# RADIOLOGIC CLINICS
## OF NORTH AMERICA

## Advances in Gastrointestinal Imaging

*Guest Editor*
LAURA R. CARUCCI, MD

March 2007 • Volume 45 • Number 2

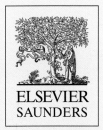

ELSEVIER
SAUNDERS

An imprint of Elsevier, Inc
PHILADELPHIA LONDON TORONTO MONTREAL SYDNEY TOKYO

**W.B. SAUNDERS COMPANY**
*A Division of Elsevier Inc.*

1600 John F. Kennedy Boulevard • Suite 1800 • Philadelphia, Pennsylvania 19103-2899

http://www.theclinics.com

**RADIOLOGIC CLINICS OF NORTH AMERICA Volume 45, Number 2**
**March 2007 ISSN 0033-8389, ISBN 1-4160-4363-2; 978-1-4160-4363-8**

*Editor:* Barton Dudlick

*Reprints:* For copies of 100 or more, of articles in this publication, please contact the Commercial Reprints Department, Elsevier Inc., 360 Park Avenue South, New York, New York 10010-1710. Tel.: (+1) 212-633-3813; Fax: (+1) 212-462-1935; E-mail: reprints@elsevier.com.

The ideas and opinions expressed in *Radiologic Clinics of North America* do not necessarily reflect those of the Publisher does not assume any responsibility for any injury and/or damage to persons or property arising out of or related to any use of the material contained in this periodical. The reader is advised to check the appropriate medical literature and the product information currently provided by the manufacturer of each drug to be administered to verify the dosage, the method and duration of administration, or contraindications, It is the responsibility of the treating physician or other health care professional, relying on independent experience and knowledge of the patient, to determine drug dosages and the best treatment for the patient. Mention of any product in this issue should not be construed as endorsement by the contributiors, editors, or the Publisher of the productor manufacturers' claims.

*Radiologic Clinics of North America* (ISSN 0033-8389) is published bimonthly in January, March, May, July, September, and November by Elsevier Inc., 360 Park Avenue South, New York, NY 10010-1710. Business and editorial offices: 1600 John F. Kenedy Boulevard, Suite 1800, Philadelphia, Pennsylvania 19103-2899. Customer Service Office: 6277 Sea Harbor Drive, Orlando, FL 32887-4800. Periodicals postage paid at New York, NY, and additional mailing offices. Subscription prices are USD 259 per year for US individuals, USD 385 per year for US institutions, USD 127 per year for US students and residents, USD 303 per year for Canadian individuals, USD 473 per year of Canadian institutions, USD 352 per year for international individuals, USD 473 per year for international institutions, and USD 171 per year for Canadian and foreign students/residents. To receive student and resident rate, orders must be accompanied by name of affiliated institution, date of term, and the signature of program/residency coordinatior on institution letterhead. Orders will be billed at individual rate until proof of status is received. Foreign air speed delivery is included in all Clinics subscriptionprices. All prices are subject to change without notice. **POSTMASTER:** Send address changes to *Radiologic Clinics of North America,* Elsevier Periodicals Customer Service, 6277 Sea Harbor Drive, Orlando, FL 32887-4800. **Customer Service: 1-800-654-2452 (US). From outside of the US, call (+1) 407-345-4000.**

*Radiologic Clinics of North America* also published in Greek Paschalidis Medical Publications, Athens, Greece.

*Radiologic Clinics of North America* is covered in *Index Medicus, EMBASE/Excerpta Medica, Current Contents/Life Sciences, Current Contents/Clinical Medicine, RSNA Index to Imaging Literature, BIOSIS, Science Citation Index,* and *ISI/BIOMED.*

Printed in the United States of America.

## GOAL STATEMENT

The goal of the *Radiologic Clinics of North America* is to keep practicing radiologists and radiology residents up to date with current clinical practice in radiology by providing timely articles reviewing the state of the art in patient care.

## ACCREDITATION

The *Radiologic Clinics of North America* is planned and implemented in accordance with the Essential Areas and Policies of the Accreditation Council for Continuing Medical Education (ACCME) through the joint sponsorship of the University of Virginia School of Medicine and Elsevier. The University of Virginia School of Medicine is accredited by the ACCME to provide continuing medical education for physicians.

The University of Virginia School of Medicine designates this educational activity for a maximum of 15 *AMA PRA Category 1 Credits*™. Physicians should only claim credit commensurate with the extent of their participation in the activity.

The American Medical Association has determined that physicians not licensed in the US who participate in this CME activity are eligible for 15 *AMA PRA Category 1 Credits*™.

Credit can be earned by reading the text material, taking the CME examination online at http://www.theclinics.com/home/cme, and completing the evaluation. After taking the test, you will be required to review any and all incorrect answers. Following completion of the test and evaluation, your credit will be awarded and you may print your certificate.

## FACULTY DISCLOSURE/CONFLICT OF INTEREST

The University of Virginia School of Medicine, as an ACCME accredited provider, endorses and strives to comply with the Accreditation Council for Continuing Medical Education (ACCME) Standards of Commercial Support, Commonwealth of Virginia statutes, University of Virginia policies and procedures, and associated federal and private regulations and guidelines on the need for disclosure and monitoring of proprietary and financial interests that may affect the scientific integrity and balance of content delivered in continuing medical education activities under our auspices.

The University of Virginia School of Medicine requires that all CME activities accredited through this institution be developed independently and be scientifically rigorous, balanced and objective in the presentation/discussion of its content, theories and practices.

All authors/editors participating in an accredited CME activity are expected to disclose to the readers relevant financial relationships with commercial entities occurring within the past 12 months (such as grants or research support, employee, consultant, stock holder, member of speakers bureau, etc.). The University of Virginia School of Medicine will employ appropriate mechanisms to resolve potential conflicts of interest to maintain the standards of fair and balanced education to the reader. Questions about specific strategies can be directed to the Office of Continuing Medical Education, University of Virginia School of Medicine, Charlottesville, Virginia.

*The authors/editors listed below have identified no financial or professional relationships for themselves or their spouse/partner:*
Rizwan Aslam, MBChB; Laura R. Carucci, MD (Guest Editor); Barton Dudlick (Acquisitions Editor); Elliott K. Fishman, MD; Amy K. Hara, MD; Karen M. Horton, MD; James E. Huprich, MD; Sonja Kinner, MD; Luis A. Landeras, MD; John C. Lappas, MD; Thomas C. Lauenstein, MD; Martina Morin, MD, FFRRCSI, FRCP; Scott R. Paulsen, MD; Richard A. Szucs, MD; Mary Ann Turner, MD; Raul N. Uppot, MD; and Jinxing Yu, MD.

*The authors/editors listed below have identified the following financial or professional relationships for themselves or their spouse/partner:*
**Abraham H. Dachman, MD, FACR** is a consultant for EZEM, Inc., iCAD, Inc., and GE Healthcare.
**Jeff Fidler, MD** receives research support from EZEM and is on the Advisory Committee/Board for General Electric.
**Stefaan Gryspeerdt, MD** serves as a consultant for EZEM and Vital Images.
**David H. Kim, MD** receives honoraria from Viatronix, and is on the Advisory Committee for CBFleet.
**Philippe Lefere, MD** serves as a consultant for EZEM and Vital Images.
**Dean D.T. Maglinte, MD** is a consultant for Cook, Inc., and EZEM, Inc.
**Perry J. Pickhardt, MD** is a consultant for Viatronix, Inc., Fleet Pharmaceutical, and Medicsight.
**Kumaresan Sandrasegaran, MD** is on the speaker's bureau for Philips Medical Systems.
**Judy Yee, MD** receives a research grant from GE Healthcare.

*Disclosure of Discussion of Non-FDA Approved Uses for Pharmaceutical and/or Medical Devices:*
**The University of Virginia School of Medicine, as an ACCME provider, requires that all authors identify and disclose any "off label" uses for pharmaceutical and medical device products. The University of Virginia School of Medicine recommends that each physician fully review all the available data on new products or procedures prior to clinical use.**

## TO ENROLL

To enroll in the *Radiologic Clinics of North America* Continuing Medical Education program, call customer service at 1-800-654-2452 or sign up online at http://www.theclinics.com/home/cme. The CME program is available to subscribers for an additional annual fee of $205.00.

## THE CLINICS ARE NOW AVAILABLE ONLINE!

Access your subscription at:
**www.theclinics.com**

# ADVANCES IN GASTROINTESTINAL IMAGING

## GUEST EDITOR

**LAURA R. CARUCCI, MD**
Associate Professor, Director of MRI, and Director
of Abdominal MR, Abdominal Imaging Section,
Department of Radiology, Virginia Commonwealth
University Medical Center, Richmond, Virginia

## CONTRIBUTORS

**RIZWAN ASLAM, MBChB**
Assistant Clinical Professor of Radiology,
Department of Radiology, University of California
San Francisco; and Staff Radiologist, Department of
Radiology, Veterans Affairs Medical Center,
San Francisco, California

**LAURA R. CARUCCI, MD**
Associate Professor, Director of MRI, and Director
of Abdominal MR, Abdominal Imaging Section,
Department of Radiology, Virginia Commonwealth
University Medical Center, Richmond, Virginia

**ABRAHAM H. DACHMAN, MD, FACR**
Department of Radiology, The University of
Chicago, Chicago, Illinois

**JEFF FIDLER, MD**
Assistant Clinical Professor and Consultant,
Department of Radiology, May Clinic, Rochester,
Minnesota

**ELLIOT K. FISHMAN, MD**
Professor of Radiology and Oncology; and Director
of Diagnostic Radiology and Body CT,
Johns Hopkins Medical Institutions,
Baltimore, Maryland

**STEFAAN GRYSPEERDT, MD**
Department of Radiology, Stedelijk Ziekenhuis,
Roselare, Belgium

**AMY A. HARA, MD**
Associate Professor, Department of Diagnostic
Radiology, Mayo Clinic Arizona, Scottsdale,
Arizona

**KAREN M. HORTON, MD**
Associate Professor of Radiology, Johns Hopkins
Medical Institutions, Baltimore, Maryland

**JAMES E. HUPRICH, MD**
Assistant Professor, Department of Diagnostic
Radiology, Mayo Clinic Rochester, Rochester,
Minnesota

**DAVID H. KIM, MD**
Department of Radiology, University of Wisconsin
Medical School, Clinical Science Center,
Madison, Wisconsin

**SONJA KINNER, MD**
Department of Radiology and Neuroradiology,
University Hospital, Essen, Germany

**LUIS A. LANDERAS, MD**
Assistant Clinical Professor of Radiology,
Department of Radiology, University of California
San Francisco; and Staff Radiologist, Department of
Radiology, Veterans Affairs Medical Center,
San Francisco, California

**JOHN C. LAPPAS, MD**
Professor of Radiology, Department of Radiology,
Wishard Memorial Hospital, Indiana University
School of Medicine, Indianapolis, Indiana

**THOMAS C. LAUENSTEIN, MD**
Assistant Professor of Radiology, Department of
Radiology and Neuroradiology, University
Hospital, Essen, Germany; Department of
Radiology, Emory University Hospital, The Emory
Clinic, Atlanta, Georgia

**PHILIPPE LEFERE, MD**
Department of Radiology, Stedelijk Ziekenhuis, Roselare, Belgium

**DEAN D.T. MAGLINTE, MD**
Professor of Radiology, Indiana University School of Medicine; and Department of Radiology, Indiana University Hospital, Indianapolis, Indiana

**MARTINA MORIN, MD, FFRRCSI, FRCR**
Department of Radiology, Beaumont Hospital, Dublin, Ireland

**SCOTT R. PAULSEN, MD**
Resident, Department of Diagnostic Radiology, Mayo Clinic Rochester, Rochester, Minnesota

**PERRY J. PICKHARDT, MD**
Department of Radiology, University of Wisconsin Medical School, Clinical Science Center, Madison, Wisconsin

**KUMARESAN SANDRASEGARAN, MD**
Assistant Professor of Radiology, Department of Radiology, Indiana University School of Medicine, Indianapolis, Indiana

**RICHARD A. SZUCS, MD**
Assistant Clinical Professor, Department of Radiology, Virginia Commonwealth University Medical Center; and Commonwealth Radiology, Bon Secours St. Mary's Hospital, Richmond, Virginia

**MARY ANN TURNER, MD**
Professor and Vice Chairman of Faculty, Department of Radiology, Abdominal Imaging Section, Virginia Commonwealth University Medical Center, Richmond, Virginia

**RAUL N. UPPOT, MD**
Assistant Radiologist and Instructor in Radiology, Division of Abdominal Imaging and Interventional Radiology, Department of Radiology, Massachusetts General Hospital, Harvard Medical School, Boston, Massachusetts

**JUDY YEE, MD**
Professor of Radiology, Department of Radiology, University of California San Francisco; and Chief of Radiology, Department of Radiology, Veterans Affairs Medical Center, San Francisco, California

**JINXING YU, MD**
Associate Professor, Abdominal Imaging Section, Department of Radiology, Virginia Commonwealth University Medical Center, Richmond, Virginia

# ADVANCES IN GASTROINTESTINAL IMAGING

Volume 45 · Number 2 · March 2007

# Contents

procedures often are performed fluoroscopically, the radiologist may play a direct role in the management of weight loss in patients following LAGB.

## Multidetector CT and MR of the Small Bowel and Mesentery

Multidetector CT is an ideal tool for the diagnosis of acute and chronic mesenteric ischemia. Advanced CT scanners and expertise in three-dimensional imaging are becoming increasingly widespread, opening the door to new opportunities and challenges in the evaluation of patients suspected of having mesenteric ischemia. This article reviews contrast administration and image acquisition protocols, the anatomy of the mesenteric vasculature, the etiology of acute and chronic mesenteric ischemia, and CT findings diagnostic for these conditions.

CT enteroclysis overcomes the individual deficiencies of both barium enteroclysis and conventional CT and combines the advantages of both into one technique whose clinical applicability has been simplified and made more reliable with multidetector CT technology. This article examines the techniques of CT enteroclysis and presents an overview of its clinical applications relative to other methods of small bowel imaging.

CT enterography (CTE) is a noninvasive imaging test using neutral intraluminal contrast and intravenous contrast to evaluate the small bowel. Multiphasic imaging is used in evaluating obscure gastrointestinal bleeding (OGIB), and single-phase enteric imaging is used for all other indications, including Crohn's disease (CD). CTE findings of CD include bowel wall thickening, mucosal hyperenhancement, and mural stratification. CTE findings of angiodyplasias include a vascular tuft visible during arterial phase and an early draining mesenteric vein. Early studies indicate that CTE is superior to barium examination in the evaluation of CD and is complementary to capsule endoscopy in the evaluation of OGIB.

Cross-sectional imaging techniques such as CT and MR imaging have advantages over traditional barium fluoroscopic techniques in their ability to visualize superimposed bowel loops better and to improve visualization of extraluminal findings and complications. This article discusses MR imaging of the small bowel with enterography and enteroclysis techniques. It reviews the advantages, limitations, technique, and indications and reviews the results that have been obtained in evaluating different disease processes.

*CT and MR Colonography (Virtual Colonoscopy)*

*Luis A. Landeras, Rizwan Aslam, and Judy Yee*

Virtual colonoscopy (VC) has acquired an important role in evaluation of the colon. In some situations it may be a safer method to visualize the colon effectively, or it may be the only available option when other techniques have failed. This article reviews state-of-the art VC technique and the results of current performance trials. It discusses the rationale for using various colonic cleansing regimens for VC. It also discusses the two distending agents for VC (room air and carbon dioxide) and presents practical tips for administration and the role of antispasmodic drugs.

*Abraham H. Dachman, Philippe Lefere, Stefaan Gryspeerdt, and Martina Morin*

Virtual colonoscopy interpretation is improving rapidly with the development of efficient software using two-dimensional, three-dimensional (3D) endoluminal, and 3D novel views such as those that seem to cut the colon open and lay it flat for interpretation. Comparison of these various views, comparisons of supine and prone positioning, and comparisons of lung and soft tissue windows aid in the recognition of various pitfalls of interpretation.

*Perry J. Pickhardt and David H. Kim*

CT colonography (CTC), also known as virtual colonoscopy, is a minimally invasive test for the detection of colorectal polyps and masses. At the authors' institution, asymptomatic screening has been the overwhelming indication for CTC referral since local third-party coverage was initiated in April 2004. This practical review details the authors' current approach to CTC screening, which has evolved and matured over time. It discusses the entire spectrum from program set-up through patient disposition following CTC examination. The authors hope this article will provide a roadmap for radiologists who wish to institute a CTC screening program.

*Sonja Kinner and Thomas C. Lauenstein*

Combining the advantages of unsurpassed soft tissue contrast and lack of ionizing radiation, MR imaging of the gastrointestinal tract has become increasingly used clinically. Both bowel inflammation and tumor disease of the large bowel can be well visualized by means of MR colonography (MRC). This article describes current techniques of MRC and gives an overview of its clinical outcome. Special focus is directed toward the evaluation of patients' acceptance of MRC.

RADIOLOGIC
CLINICS
OF NORTH AMERICA

Radiol Clin N Am 45 (2007) xi–xii

# Preface

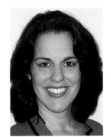

Laura R. Carucci, MD
*Department of Radiology*
*Virginia Commonwealth University Medical Center*
*1250 E. Marshall Street*
*Richmond, VA 23298, USA*

*E-mail address:*
lcarucci@vcu.edu

Laura R. Carucci, MD
*Guest Editor*

This issue of the *Radiologic Clinics of North America* is devoted to advances in gastrointestinal imaging. It is divided into three sections focusing on areas that are interesting and challenging in gastrointestinal imaging: imaging of obesity and following bariatric surgery, multidetector CT and MR imaging of the small bowel, and multidetector CT and MRI imaging of the colon (virtual colonoscopy). This issue reviews recent technologic advances and provides a resource for the performance and interpretation of these advances in both academic and general practice.

The first section is devoted to imaging of obesity and imaging after bariatric surgery. The prevalence of obesity is increasing in epidemic proportions, and the impact of this condition has direct and dramatic effects on the practice of radiology, particularly in the field of abdominal imaging. Therefore, it is important for radiologists to be aware of the various bariatric procedures performed and their associated complications. This section includes articles that address the impact of obesity on radiology and imaging after the popular bariatric surgical procedures of adjustable laparoscopic gastric banding and Roux-en-Y gastric bypass surgery.

The next section covers cross-sectional imaging of the small bowel using the techniques of multidetector CT and MR imaging. The evaluation of mesenteric ischemia using multidetector CT angiography is reviewed, as are techniques and applications for CT enteroclysis and CT enterography. Special attention is directed toward CT enterography for Crohn's disease and occult upper gastrointestinal bleeding. In addition, MR imaging of the small bowel is discussed in detail.

The final section reviews CT and MR colonography. The first article describes CT colonography (virtual colonoscopy) with emphasis on procedural techniques and efficacy. The second article regarding CT colonography provides valuable information on visualization methodology, interpretation, and potential pitfalls. The next article presents a practical guide for developing a successful virtual colonoscopy screening program. The final article of the section discusses the intriguing topic of MR colonography.

I thank Dr. Frank Miller for his assistance in developing this project and Barton Dudlick and the W.B. Saunders Company for the opportunity to create this issue of the *Radiologic Clinics of North America*. I am extremely grateful to the authors whose dedication and expertise made this issue possible. I wish to thank my husband, Dr. Adam Klausner, for his unwavering support, Dr. Mary Ann Turner and Dr. Ann Fulcher for their guidance, and Dr. Marc Levine for training me to be an academic radiologist. Finally, I wish to dedicate this issue to Dr. Igor Laufer, my mentor and friend, who inspired my career and taught me to appreciate the art of gastrointestinal radiology.

RADIOLOGIC
CLINICS
OF NORTH AMERICA

Radiol Clin N Am 45 (2007) 231–246

**ELSEVIER
SAUNDERS**

# Impact of Obesity on Radiology

Raul N. Uppot, MD

Obesity is impacting radiology departments throughout the country. Increasingly, the ability to acquire and interpret images is compromised by a patient's body habitus. A recent study demonstrated that the number of radiology studies considered difficult to interpret as a result of patient obesity has doubled over the course of 15 years [1]. Because of an increased incidence of diabetes, heart disease, and certain forms of cancer [2], the direct impact of obesity on overall health is well known; however, obesity also impacts health in more indirect ways. In this regard, delivery of

The author has served as a consultant for Siemens Medical Solutions and was paid to write a MRI Hot Topic Internal Siemens paper in 2005 titled, "MRI Hot Topics Obesity and MR Imaging."
Division of Abdominal Imaging and Interventional Radiology, Department of Radiology, Massachusetts General Hospital, Harvard Medical School, 55 Fruit Street, White #270, Boston, MA 02114, USA
*E-mail address:* ruppot@partners.org

doi:10.1016/j.rcl.2007.03.001

quality health care may be compromised in areas such as safe patient transport [3,4], the ability to render diagnoses based on physical examination [5,6] or medical imaging [1,7–11], and the ability to provide adequate treatment for patients within a health care facility [12–16]. Two factors responsible for the current crisis in medical imaging as a result of obesity are (1) the rising prevalence of obesity in the United States and around the world, and (2) the increasing popularity of bariatric surgery such as gastric bypass surgery, leading to an acute influx of morbidly obese patients into hospitals. Until now, radiologists have not been particularly attuned to obesity. Obesity is a metabolic health issue not diagnosed by radiologists. Because of its growing impact on image acquisition and quality, obesity is now an issue that needs to be examined and addressed by the medical imaging community.

This article (1) provides radiologists with background information about obesity including the definition of obesity, the prevalence of obesity, and the health and economic implications; (2) describes current problems and provides specific solutions related to imaging obese patients using various modalities; and (3) discusses the future of medical imaging and obesity.

## Background

### Definition of obesity

Obesity is not defined simply by body weight. Since the 1800s, obesity has been defined by body mass index (BMI). BMI, first described by Belgian scientist Adolphe Quetelet in 1830, represents a statistical measure of the weight of an individual scaled according to height and is measured in $kg/m^2$.

Physicians use the BMI as an estimate of total body fat [17,18]. Current BMI classifications in $kg/m^2$ are as follows: BMI less than 18.5, underweight; BMI 18.5 to 24.9, normal weight; BMI 25.0 to 29.9, overweight; BMI greater than 30, obese; and BMI greater than 40, morbidly obese. Recent articles, however, question the validity of the BMI to estimate total body fat [19,20]. From an imaging perspective, an individual's diameter and body weight is more important than total body fat or BMI [21]. Imaging equipment is designed for a set body diameter and body weight, and if patients exceed these limits, they cannot be imaged.

### Prevalence of obesity

The prevalence of obesity is increasing in the United States and throughout the world. Currently, more than 60 million Americans adults (>20 years old) have a BMI greater than 30 $kg/m^2$ [2]. Overall, 66% of Americans are overweight, obese, or morbidly obese [2], and currently 6 million individuals are considered morbidly obese with a BMI greater than 40 $kg/m^2$. The prevalence of morbid obesity has increased from 0.8 % in 1960 to 2.9% in 1988 to 4.7% in 2000 [22]. The prevalence of obesity has increased progressively in every state (Fig. 1). Although most obese patients can be imaged adequately, the difficulty in acquiring diagnostic quality images increases as the degree of obesity increases, and larger patients may not fit on imaging equipment.

In addition to the rising prevalence of obesity, the increased prevalence of bariatric surgery is leading to an influx of obese patients into health centers throughout the country. Gastric bypass surgery has become the surgical treatment of choice for the

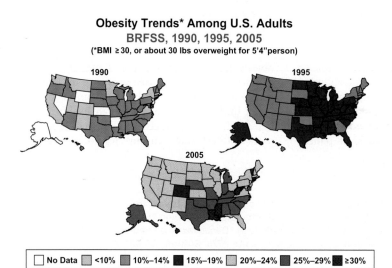

**Obesity Trends\* Among U.S. Adults**
BRFSS, 1990, 1995, 2005
(\*BMI ≥ 30, or about 30 lbs overweight for 5'4"person)

1990    1995

2005

☐ No Data  ☐ <10%  ■ 10%–14%  ■ 15%–19%  ☐ 20%–24%  ■ 25%–29%  ■ ≥30%

*Fig. 1.* Obesity trends in the United State by state in 1990, 1995, and 2005. There is a progressive increase in the prevalence of obesity from 1990 to 2005. (*From* Centers for Disease Control and Prevention. Behavioral risk factor surveillance system. Available at: http://www.cdc.gov/nccdphp/dnpa/obesity/trend/maps. Accessed April 6, 2007.)

management of morbid obesity in the United States, and the number of gastric bypass surgeries performed in the United States has increased from 67,000 in 2002 to 140,000 in 2005 [23–25].

The impact of bariatric surgery on medical imaging is apparent. Healthy morbidly obese patients who previously would not have needed hospital care now are being hospitalized for this surgery and its potential complications. The impact of this patient influx on radiology departments occurs from the moment these patients enter the hospital, because they typically require a preoperative ultrasound and a postoperative upper gastrointestinal examination. Difficulty in imaging this group of patients becomes more serious when they develop complications and either no imaging modality is available to evaluate them, or the image quality is severely limited.

## Impact of obesity on health and delivery of health care

Obesity has been linked to various clinical conditions including type 2 diabetes, hypertension, heart disease, and certain forms of cancer such as endometrial, colon, and breast cancer [2]. Obesity stresses the body with a greater strain on cardiac output and increased wear and tear on joints leading to osteoarthritis [2]. In addition to its direct impact on health, obesity increasingly is understood to have an indirect impact on health by affecting the delivery of health care. Difficulties in managing obese patients within a health care facility have been documented. Obese patients require larger wheelchairs, larger doors, larger beds, and larger operating room tables (Fig. 2) [3,4]. The ability to perform an adequate clinical examination is compromised

also [5,6], because it becomes difficult to listen to heart sounds, lung respiration, and bowel sounds. In addition, the ability to palpate the abdomen, perform a pelvic examination, and evaluate for masses is compromised.

## Obesity and the radiology department

The impact of obesity on radiology departments is multifactorial. Obesity can affect the throughput of the department. Obesity limits the ability of patients to fit on existing imaging equipment and the ability to acquire and interpret images adequately. Furthermore, to obtain quality images in obese patients, an increased radiation dose may be required. Difficulties also arise in patient positioning and access for image-guided interventional procedures. There is potential for injury to technologists and transport crew when moving and positioning patients. Moreover, there is increased wear and tear on imaging equipment, with faster tube burn out and stress on table motors [1].

### Scheduling/transportation/throughput

Knowing a patient's weight and body diameter is important before scheduling a patient for an imaging examination. All medical imaging equipment has standard weight and bore/gantry diameter limits. Individuals scheduling a patient must know the patient's weight and diameter and confirm that they do not exceed the specifications of the available imaging equipment. In addition, accommodations must be made to ensure that the appropriate transportation resources (larger beds, larger wheelchairs, adequate nursing and transport

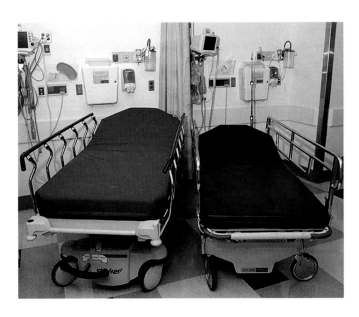

Fig. 2. Larger bariatric transport bed (*left*) compared with normal-sized transportation bed (*right*). Efficiency in the transport of obese patients to the radiology department depends on the availability and number of these larger bariatric beds.

crew) are available to bring the patient at the scheduled time. The throughput of a busy radiology department can be disrupted if a scheduled obese patient cannot be brought to the department or cannot fit on imaging equipment. The obese patient's study must be postponed or cancelled, and this situation also may increase waiting time and frustration for other patients.

### Cancelled cases

When nondiagnostic images are acquired or when a case is cancelled because the patient cannot fit on imaging equipment, clinical and economic issues arise. At our institution, three outcomes have been observed for patients who could not fit on imaging equipment. First, they may be referred to an outpatient imaging facility with an open MR imaging scanner that can accommodate larger patients. This option has limitations, however, because not all conditions can be diagnosed using MR imaging, not all patients can tolerate MR imaging, and the image quality of open MR imaging tends to be lower than cylindrical-bore MR imaging because of lower gradient strengths. Second, they may be admitted and clinically observed. Serial in-hospital clinical and laboratory examinations sometimes may aid the diagnosis of a condition, but there are economic implications because there are increased costs associated with longer hospital stays and further laboratory testing. Third, they may undergo exploratory surgery. On rare occasions, when a patient has an acute medical condition that cannot be diagnosed with medical imaging, exploratory surgery may be required. The difficulty with this option is that surgery in obese patients is technically more difficult, and there is potential for increased morbidity and mortality.

In the past several years imaging equipment manufactures have begun to address the issue of obesity. Many manufacturers have increased the available table weight limits and aperture diameters to accommodate larger patients. Given the increasing prevalence of obesity in the United States, manufacturers and imaging facilities that directly address the issue of obesity may capture a niche market in medical imaging.

Obesity affects each imaging modality differently. For CT, MR imaging, and fluoroscopy the primary limitation is whether the patient can fit on the imaging equipment (Table 1). For ultrasound, plain radiographs, and nuclear medicine, attenuation through excessive fat is an important limitation. Of all imaging modalities, ultrasound is most directly limited by obesity [1]. If a patient can fit on CT equipment, then CT is the preferred imaging modality in the obese patient. Limitations and

**Table 1:** Maximal available weight limit and aperture diameter per imaging modality

| Imaging modality | Weight limit (lb) | Maximum aperture diameter (cm) |
|---|---|---|
| Fluoroscopy | 700 | 63 |
| Multidetector CT | 680 | 90 |
| Cylindrical-bore MR imaging 1.5 T | 550 | 70 |
| Vertical-field MR imaging 0.3–1.0 T | 550 | 55 |

solutions associated with each imaging modality are addressed separately in the following sections.

## Ultrasound

The effects of obesity on ultrasound begin to be seen at weights of 250 to 300 lbs. Although ultrasound has the advantage of being performed portably and therefore is not limited by table weight or aperture diameter, it is compromised by fat attenuation, a small footprint, and difficulties in patient positioning.

### Fat attenuation

Ultrasound beams are attenuated by fat, and this attenuation limits image quality (Fig. 3). The attenuation coefficient of fat for sound is 0.63 dB/cm at 1 MHz, and therefore, as the thickness of subcutaneous fat increases or as the frequency of the transducer increases, the attenuation of the ultrasound beam increases. It is difficult, however, to predict reliably the degree of fat attenuation and the resultant image quality in an obese patient. Some obese patients will have excellent image quality, whereas others will have nondiagnostic examinations. There are two reasons for this unpredictability in predetermining the sonographic image quality: (1) the attenuation of ultrasound beams by soft tissues, which varies greatly among individuals independent of the thickness of the soft tissues, and (2) differences in the distribution of fat. The distribution of subcutaneous, intraperitoneal, and retroperitoneal fat can play a significant role in determining the thickness of the fat that the ultrasound beam must penetrate (Fig. 4). For example, two 300-lb patients who present for hepatic sonography may have different image quality. The patient who weighs 300 lb and has predominantly subcutaneous fat has a larger depth to reach the liver parenchyma and will have worse image quality than the 300-lb patient who has a negligible depth of subcutaneous fat and predominately intraperitoneal fat.

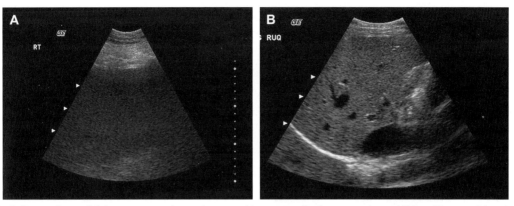

*Fig. 3.* Comparison of right upper quadrant ultrasound image quality in two patients. (*A*) In a 45-year-old patient weighing 250 lb, ultrasound images are nondiagnostic. (*B*) In a 45-year-old patient weighing 150 lb, ultrasound images show normal liver parenchyma.

Renal sonograms also are limited if there is a predominance of perinephric fat.

### Footprint

The ultrasound footprint represents the surface area of the probe that abuts the skin surface. The larger the foot print, the larger the surface area that is covered and imaged. At our institution, a transducer with a bandwidth of 1.5 to 4.5 MHz that has a footprint of 61 × 17 mm is used.

### Patient positioning

Ultrasound is operator dependent, and proper patient positioning plays an important role in acquiring quality images. The difficulty in turning noncooperative obese patients in oblique, lateral, and prone positions can be a limiting factor (Fig. 5). In addition, difficulties in properly

positioning obese patients can lead to injuries for technologists [26].

### Specific solutions

Depth of ultrasound penetration may be improved by using the lowest-frequency transducer. Abdominal ultrasound of obese patients should be performed with transducers that have a frequency of 1.5 to 2 MHz. Lower frequencies, however, result in decreased axial and lateral image resolution. Use of harmonics may improve penetration and image quality [27]. A harmonic signal is generated when the primary ultrasound beam extending through a depth of tissue expands and compresses the tissues. These tissues subsequently generate sound at a frequency two to three times the frequency of the primary beam. Ultrasound units can filter electronically and detect only the

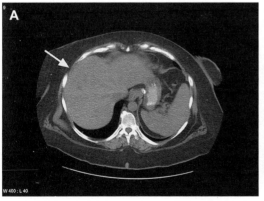

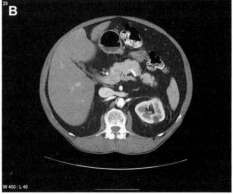

*Fig. 4.* Axial abdominal CT images in two different 300-1b patients comparing the distribution of body fat. (*A*) Axial CT at the level of the liver shows the thickness of subcutaneous fat (*arrow*), which may limit an ultrasound examination. (*B*) Axial CT at the level of the liver shows a paucity of subcutaneous fat but a prominence of intraperitoneal fat. The thickness of the subcutaneous tissues is minimal and would not limit an ultrasound examination. (*From* Uppot RN, Sahani DV, Hahn PF, et al. Impact of obesity on medical imaging and image-guided intervention. AJR Am J Roentgenol 2007;188(2):433–40; with permission from the American Journal of Roentgenology.)

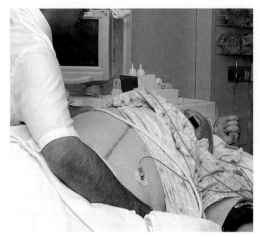

*Fig. 5.* Operator difficulties in patient access and positioning for an ultrasound examination.

harmonic frequency, resulting in a better signal-to-noise ratio and improved contrast and spatial resolution. Theoretically, because a greater depth is necessary for generation of the harmonics, harmonic imaging may be more useful in larger patients. Studies comparing harmonics with conventional ultrasound in hepatic sonography showed no correlation between image quality and body habitus [28].

Image quality also may be improved by decreasing the depth to the target organ. Poor penetration of the ultrasound beam beyond the focal depth results in poor image quality. Images beyond 8 to 10 cm of depth become uninterpretable. To achieve the shortest distance to the target organ, the following strategies may be used:

1. Review any prior cross-sectional imaging to determine the shortest distance to the organ of interest, and position the patient so that the organ of interest is at the shortest possible distance from the transducer.
2. Use pillows and splints to position patients.
3. Use the liver–spleen window to image the kidneys.
4. Apply pressure on the probe to displace the subcutaneous fat and decrease the distance to the target organ.

## CT

Multidetector CT (MDCT) is the modality of choice to image obese patients because it allows rapid image acquisition, high resolution with isotropic voxels, and off-axis reformations. The patient must be able to fit in the scanner, however, and limitations in MDCT image quality resulting from obesity have been reported, particularly for chest CT for

pulmonary embolism [7] and positron emission tomography CT [10].

## Is fat good for multidetector CT?

MDCT imaging of the internal organs is aided by an abundance of intraperitoneal fat because it tends to separate bowel loops and internal organs, allowing improved visualization (Fig. 6). CT is not useful, however, if the patient cannot fit into the scanner. Whether a patient can fit depends on table weight and gantry diameter limits. Most institutions with 16- or 64-slice MDCT scanners have table weights limits of 450 lb and gantry diameter limits of 70 cm. Newer MDCT scanners have increased table weights and gantry diameters up to 680 lb and 90 cm, respectively.

## Table weight

Although technically the CT table itself can withstand weights greater than 700 lb, the limitations for the table exist because of the table motor. The table motor must be able to raise the patient and move the table into the gantry at a constant speed. Manufacturing standards dictate that tables must be able to distribute the load, and the motor must be able to move the table into the gantry at a consistent speed to an accuracy of 0.25 mm. Designing motors that can manage a large weight load with 0.25 mm accuracy is the challenge in designing equipment for obese patients. The challenge is potentially even greater in faster, 64-slice MDCT because it requires increasing the table motor speed while maintaining accuracy with a heavy load.

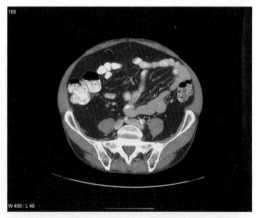

*Fig. 6.* Axial CT in a 56-year-old man with extensive intra-abdominal mesenteric fat shows separation of the small bowel mesentery and internal organs allowing better visualization. (*From* Uppot RN, Sahani DV, Hahn PF, et al. Impact of obesity on medical imaging and image-guided intervention. AJR Am J Roentgenol 2007;188(2):439; with permission from the American Journal of Roentgenology.)

## Gantry diameter

The standard gantry diameter for MDCT is approximately 70 cm. This dimension represents the horizontal diameter of the CT gantry. A more clinically relevant measurement is the vertical diameter with the table in the gantry. When the table apparatus is advanced into the gantry, the vertical diameter decreases by 15 to 18 cm, further limiting the size of the patient that may be imaged (Fig. 7). Therefore, for most CT equipment, the true available diameter for a patient placed supine is 52 to 55 cm. Larger-diameter gantries have been used for many years for radiation treatment planning in radiation oncology departments. The diagnostic quality of these CT images was limited by greater source-to-image distance. In recent years, however, manufactures have modified and improved the diagnostic quality of these larger-bore CT scanners and are now marketing them for imaging obese patients. As of this writing the largest commercially available gantry diameter for diagnostic imaging is 90 cm.

## Field of view

Enlarging the gantry diameter is of no use without an associated increase in the field of view. Standard MDCT has a field of view of 50 cm. Therefore, some patients who can fit into the scanner exceed the field of view and are imaged inadequately with artifacts, as described later. Newer, large-bore CT scanners have an extended field of view up to 82 cm [23].

## Collimation/table speed and pitch

Collimation also plays an important role in image quality. With thinner collimation, there is increased

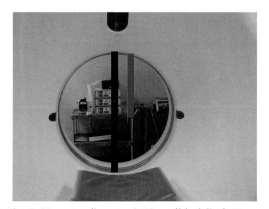

*Fig. 7.* CT gantry diameter is 70 cm (*black line*). Movement of the CT table into the gantry will decrease its vertical diameter to 55 cm (*red line*). (*From* Uppot RN, Sahani DV, Hahn PF, et al. Impact of obesity on medical imaging and image-guided intervention. AJR Am J Roentgenol 2007;188(2):434; with permission from the American Journal of Roentgenology.)

noise. Image quality may be improved in obese patients by using a thicker collimation and or by reconstructing to thicker slices to reduce the noise [29]. A slower table speed and decreased pitch also can improve image quality in obese patients.

## Kilovoltage peak/milliamperes per second/noise index

The increased quantity of soft tissue through which the X-ray beams must penetrate results in increased image noise in obese patients. For MDCT, the noise index may be adjusted based on the patient's body weight. At the author's institution, the noise index setting is as follows: for patients weighing less than 135 1b, the noise index is set at 10; for patients weighing 136 to 200 1b, the noise index is set at 12.5, and for patients weighing more than 200 1b, the noise index is set at 15. In obese patients kilovoltage peak (kVp) and milliamperes per second (mAs) need to be increased to obtain diagnostic images (Table 2). To obtain optimal images, a kVp of at least 140 is necessary to penetrate through the adipose tissue; water phantom studies using a 45-cm water phantom on a 64-slice MDCT showed that a kVp of 140 was mandatory to penetrate through a morbidly obese patient [29,30]. In addition, the equipment setting must be changed from "fixed mAs" to "automatic mAs," allowing the scanner to deliver the correct amount of amperes to image the patient (Fig. 8). Finally, the gantry rotation speed must be decreased from a standard one rotation/0.5 seconds to one rotation/1.0 seconds to increase the effective mAs.

## Artifacts

MDCT is a good choice for imaging obese patients because it provides intimate details of internal structure at a very good resolution. MDCT may be compromised by artifacts, however. Two artifacts that limit the image quality of obese patients are beam-hardening artifact and cropping. Beam-hardening artifact occurs when the patient exceeds the CT field of view (a 50-cm field of view in a 70-cm gantry) and the computer registers the peripheral

*Table 2:* Multidetector CT protocol for imaging obese patients

| MDCT parameters | Standard patient | Obese patient (> 350 1b) |
|---|---|---|
| kVp | 120 | 140 |
| mAs | fixed mAs | automatic mAs |
| Gantry rotation speed | 1 rotation/ 0.5 seconds | 1 rotation/ 1 second |
| Pitch | 1.1 | 0.6 |

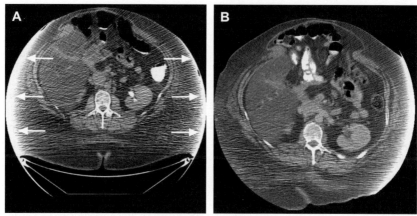

*Fig. 8.* A 39-year-old 413-1b woman. (*A*) Axial CT of the abdomen with "fixed mAs" resulted in increased noise. Beam-hardening artifact is visualized where the patient's body exceeds the field of view (*arrows*). (*B*) Repeat axial CT of the abdomen with equipment setting switched to "automatic mAs" allows the CT to increase the mAs and thereby decrease the noise. (*From* Uppot RN, Sahani DV, Hahn PF, et al. Impact of obesity on medical imaging and image-guided intervention. AJR Am J Roentgenol 2007;188(2):437; with permission from the American Journal of Roentgenology.)

edges of each image as bright attenuation (see Fig. 8). Patients who exceed the field of view also are at risk of having their images cropped by the radiologist or technologists concentrating on internal organ structures. In patients suspected of having metastasis or infections, the uncropped subcutaneous tissues must be examined to exclude pathology (Fig. 9).

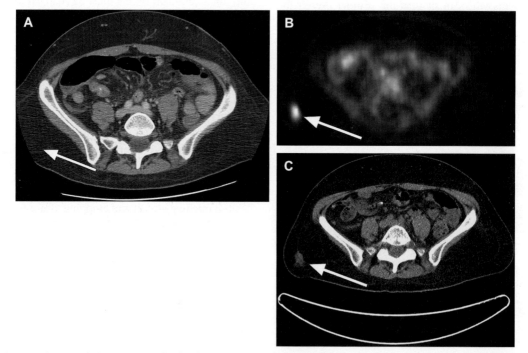

*Fig. 9.* Positron emission tomography (PET)-CT in a 52-year-old 177-1b woman with a history of carcinoid tumor. (*A*) Axial CT in a PET-CT study to look for metastasis. The CT image was cropped to focus on intra-abdominal structures (*arrow*). (*B*) PET portion of the study, which was not cropped, showed an area of fluorodeoxyglucose (FDG) uptake (*arrow*). (*C*) Review of the uncropped axial CT image showed a soft tissue deposit (*arrow*) corresponding to the area of FDG uptake seen on PET. (*From* Uppot RN, Sahani DV, Hahn PF, et al. Impact of obesity on medical imaging and image-guided intervention. AJR Am J Roentgenol 2007;188(2):437; with permission from the American Journal of Roentgenology.)

## Radiation doses in obese patients

Adjustments to the kVp and mAs made to achieve diagnostic image quality in morbidly obese patients will result in increased radiation dose. Although definite values have not been calculated, the added radiation is likely an incremental increase from the standard 8 millisievert (mSv) for chest CT and 10 mSv for abdominal/pelvic CT.

## Dual-source multidetector CT

The recent introduction of dual-source CT offers potential for improved image quality in obese patients. Studies using water phantoms show that dual-source MDCT can provide more optimal image quality in obese patients because of higher X-ray tube power (80 kW from two sources for a total of 160 kW) and data oversampling from two detector arrays [31].

## Intravenous contrast

In obese patients it often is difficult to obtain intravenous access to administer intravenous contrast for CT. The ability to obtain intravenous access may be improved by using warm compresses, displacing the adipose tissue, using anatomic landmarks, and using multiple tourniquets [16]. Although administered CT contrast doses are calculated based on cm³/kg, at the author's institution a maximum total dose of 125 cm³ iopamidol 76% is not exceeded in imaging obese patients. This maximum resulted in part because of the 450-lb weight limit of the CT equipment. With the advent of CT scanners that allow imaging of patients up to 680 lb, the total dose of intravenous contrast may need to be reassessed to opacify the internal organs adequately.

## MR imaging

The advantages of MR imaging include superior soft tissue contrast, multiplanar capabilities, and lack of ionizing radiation. For many years, vertical open-field MR imaging was the study of choice for patients who exceeded 450 1bs and 70 cm body diameter. Often, hospitals referred obese patients to open MR imaging scanners located in outpatient facilities. Both the table weight limits and aperture openings were larger with open MR units. Although open MR imaging machines exceeded the 350-1b weight limit and 60-cm diameter of closed cylindrical-bore MR imaging, they had a lower field strength (0.3–1.0 Tesla [T]) compared with standard cylindrical-bore MR imaging units (1.5–3.0 T), with resultant decreased image quality. Recent advances in cylindrical-bore technology may change the practice of outpatient referrals.

With cylindrical-bore MR equipment, there are both design and technical limitations in imaging obese patients. Design limitations include bore diameter and length, coil configurations, and table weight limit. Technical limitations include an adequate signal-to-noise ratio, field of view, scan times, and artifacts [32]. Limitations with regards to administration of intravenous contrast are similar those with CT, as discussed previously.

## MR design limitations

### Bore diameter and bore length

Bore diameter and bore length are important factors to consider when imaging obese patients with MR imaging. Bore diameter determines whether a patient can fit into the MR scanner based on patient width. Most cylindrical-bore MR scanners have a bore diameter of 60 cm (Fig. 10). As in CT, the vertical diameter is decreased when the table is positioned within the bore. Bore length is important because of claustrophobia. The longer the bore length, the more uncomfortable the MR study is for the obese or claustrophobic patient. Standard cylindrical bore lengths vary from 149 to 170 cm. Recently, manufactures have introduced cylindrical-bore 1.5-T MR imaging with larger bore

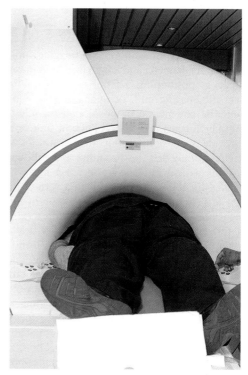

*Fig. 10.* Photograph showing cylindrical-bore MR imaging: the small MR imaging bore diameter allows limited space for the patient.

diameters (70 cm) and shorter bore lengths (125 cm) to address the issue of imaging obese patients [32].

### Coil configurations

An additional design factor to consider in MR imaging of the obese patient is the coil configuration. The highest-quality MR imaging is obtained with phased-array body coils that are placed on top of the patient as compared with the native magnet coils. The positioning of these coils further limits the available space within the bore. In fact, space constraints may preclude the use of phased-array coils. This limitation can result in suboptimal image quality. A larger bore diameter may allow the use of phased-array coils in obese patients.

### Table weight

As in CT, if a patient's weight exceeds the weight limit of the MR table, the study cannot be acquired. Exceeding the designated table weight limit impacts table motion. Open MR imaging systems have a slight advantage, because there is no dependence on table mobility. The table weight limit for open MR imaging may extend up to 550 lb, but these units have lower gradient strengths and decreased image quality. Recent advances by manufacturers of 1.5-T MR imaging scanners now allow a weight limit up to 550 lb [32].

## MR design solutions

With standard cylindrical-bore MR imaging, limitations of bore diameter and length may be addressed by patient positioning, referral to a vertical-field open MR imaging unit, or upgrading MR equipment. The patient can be positioned so only the area to be imaged is placed in the bore and/or the least wide dimension of the patient enters the MR imaging scanner first (ie, the author and colleagues place the patient into the scanner feet first when imaging the abdomen). Referral to a vertical-field open MR scanner may address the issue of table weight limit; however, the advantages in terms of aperture diameter are not as great. The vertical diameter of open MR imaging units varies from 45 to 55 cm. In addition, open MR scanners have lower gradient strengths and lower signal-to-noise ratios than cylindrical-bore MR imaging and are not as capable of advanced applications. Upgrading MR equipment may provide the best option for imaging obese patients. New 1.5-T MR imaging machines combine features of standard cylindrical-bore MR imaging (stronger gradients, higher signal-to-noise ratios, and advanced applications) with the ability to image larger patients (weight limit up to 550 lbs and bore diameter of 70 cm).

## Technical limitations of MR imaging

Technical limitations of MR imaging in obese patients are related to signal-to-noise ratios, field of view, scan times, and artifacts.

### Signal-to-noise ratio

Understanding the effects of obesity on signal-to-noise ratio is important in addressing limitations in image quality. For signal-to-noise ratio two factors need to be considered in MR imaging: the propagation of radiofrequency (RF) signal and the reception of the RF signal. Soft tissues can attenuate RF beams minimally; however, the degree of attenuation is not as great as that seen with ultrasound waves. MR surface coils can boost the RF signal that penetrates through the patient. The RF penetration depth is independent of field strength, but higher field strengths can increase the signal-to-noise ratio and improve the spectral resolution. RF heat energy deposition can occur in areas where a patient's body abuts the inner surface of the gantry and can result in minor burns. This problem is of particular concern for imaging obese patients. Receiver coils also are limited by a patient's body habitus: the inner structures of an obese patient are farther away from the receiver coils. A larger body habitus will result in increased noise and decreased contrast-to-noise ratio.

### Field of view

Larger patients require larger fields of views. There is an inverse relationship between image resolution and field of view, however, so that the larger the field of view, the lower the image resolution, and vice versa. The typical standard field of view in 1.5-T cylindrical-bore systems is 40 to 50 cm. Vertical-field open MR systems typically have lower field of views ranging from 35 to 40 cm. Ideal imaging would involve using the smallest field of view for the area of interest without inducing wrap-around artifact.

### Scan times

With regards to imaging obese patients, a larger cross-sectional area to be imaged requires an increased field of view, and a longer craniocaudal dimension requires the acquisition of more slices. These factors result in increased scan times. Longer acquisition times lead to motion artifacts.

### Artifacts

Two artifacts commonly seen in obese patients are wrap-around artifact and near-field artifact. Wrap-around artifact occurs when the area imaged exceeds the set field of view. When this circumstance occurs in the abdomen, portions of the anterior

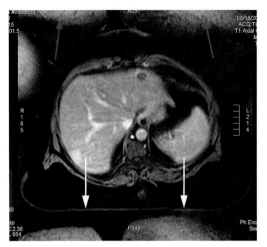

**Fig. 11.** T1-weighted fat saturated axial gadolinium-enhanced MR imaging in a 44-year-old woman. Wrap-around artifact (*white arrows*) is seen because of the small field of view. There also is inadequate fat saturation (*red arrows*) in areas where the patient's body touches the bore. (*From* Uppot RN, Sahani DV, Hahn PF, et al. Impact of obesity on medical imaging and image-guided intervention. AJR Am J Roentgenol 2007;188(2):440; with permission from the American Journal of Roentgenology.)

In areas where the patient's body abuts the bore, the RF signal propagation and receipt result in a bright signal along the periphery of the image that can interfere with evaluation of the internal organ structures.

### MR imaging technical solutions

One solution is the use of higher gradient field strengths to increase the signal-to-noise ratio and improve the spectral resolution. 3.0-T scanners may be able to provide improved image quality in obese patients. The ability to image a larger field of view is advantageous for imaging obese patients, but the larger field of view can result in decreased image resolution. Therefore, it is best to use the smallest field of view for the area of interest without inducing wrap-around artifact. In addition, noise from subcutaneous fat can be decreased by using saturation bands. Again, upgrading MR equipment provides improved imaging of obese patients. Newer MR machines using matrix coils with multiple elements combined with moving table options allow creation of a virtual field of view up to 205 cm [32].

## Plain radiographs and fluroscopy

Plain radiographs and fluoroscopy play an important role in imaging obese patients. Fluoroscopy, in particular, is used routinely to evaluate for postoperative complications after bariatric surgery.

### Table weight and aperture diameter

As with CT and MR imaging, table weight and aperture diameter are important factors to consider in imaging obese patients. The standard table weight

body are projected over the posterior body on the acquired images (Fig. 11). Wrap-around artifact can be corrected by (1) choosing the "no wrap option" on the MR scanner, (2) increasing the field of view as much as possible, and (3) changing the configuration of the field of view from rectangular to square to avoid cutoff. Near-field artifact is similar to the beam-hardening artifact visualized on CT.

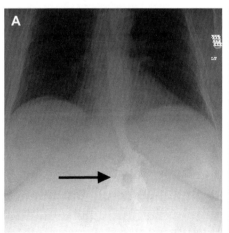
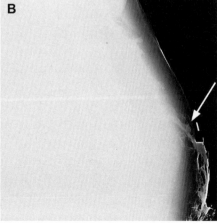

**Fig. 12.** Frontal and lateral chest radiographs performed as a substitute for a fluoroscopic gastrografin swallow in an obese patient after gastric bypass. The patient could not fit on the fluoroscopy table. (*A*) Frontal radiograph shows an enterocutaneous fistula (*arrow*). (*B*) Lateral radiograph confirms the enterocutaneous fistula (*arrow*). (*From* Uppot RN, Sahani DV, Hahn PF, et al. Impact of obesity on medical imaging and image-guided intervention. AJR Am J Roentgenol 2007;188(2):436; with permission from the American Journal of Roentgenology.)

in many institutions is 350 lb. Manufacturers are now increasing this limit up to 700 lb. The standard aperture diameter is 45 to 63 cm. At the author's institution, patients who present for an upper gastrointestinal examination following gastric bypass surgery who exceed the table weight or aperture dimensions have studies performed as serial radiographs. An initial scout radiograph is followed by multiple sequential chest radiographs as the patient swallows the oral contrast (Fig. 12). If there is a high clinical suspicion for pathology, the patient may be referred for an unenhanced CT scan, because the table weight limit of the CT scanners (450 1bs) is greater than that of the fluoroscopy tables (350 lb). Postoperative leak, fistula, or obstruction then may be assessed with CT.

### Cassette size/field of view

The film cassette size becomes an issue for acquiring film or digital radiographs in obese patients who have large surface areas. The largest standard film cassette available is 14 × 17 in (Fig. 13). Technologists who image obese patients should be aware of patient size and should consider using multiple cassettes to obtain quadrants of the patient's body rather than attempting to estimate the area of interest on a single cassette.

### Kilovoltage peak/milliamperes per second/noise

One of the biggest limitations in imaging obese patients with plain radiographs is inadequate penetration of X-ray beams resulting in increased noise and low image contrast. Also, the increased time required for penetration results in motion artifact.

Solutions to improve signal-to-noise ratio and tissue contrast for plain radiographs in obese patients include measures taken before acquiring the film as well as postacquisition measures. The use of a Bucky grid can minimize scatter. In addition, the kVp and mAs should be increased. When the author and colleagues obtain chest radiographs in obese patients, they increase the kVp from standard values of 90 to 95 kVp to 100 kVp and increase the mAs from the standard 2 to 2.5 mAs to 4 mAs (Fig. 14). After acquisition, they increase the development speed to 800. In addition, the use of digital radiography instead of film allows adjustments of the window and level to be made on the workstation monitor after image acquisition, and these adjustments may allow improved visualization of internal structures.

## Mammography

In many respects, an abundance of fatty tissue in the breast may be helpful in mammography. Internal mammary fat separates structure and provides good tissue contrast between mammary tissues and benign or malignant soft tissue nodules. Obesity poses limitations to mammography, however, that include inadequate penetration and difficulties with compression. These problems can result

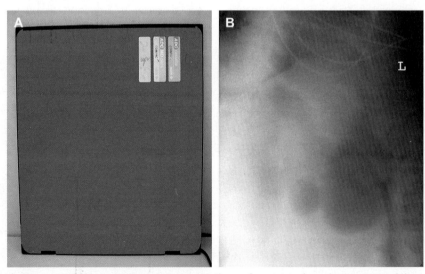

Fig. 13. Standard 14 × 17-in film cassette may not cover the surface area of an obese patient. (A) 14 × 17-in film cassette. (B) Abdominal radiograph of the left upper quadrant in an obese patient. It is more practical to obtain multiple quadrant radiographs in an obese patient rather than trying to fit the entire abdomen onto one limited-quality abdominal radiograph. (From Uppot RN, Sahani DV, Hahn PF, et al. Impact of obesity on medical imaging and image-guided intervention. AJR Am J Roentgenol 2007;188(2):433–40; with permission from the American Journal of Roentgenology.)

**A** **B**

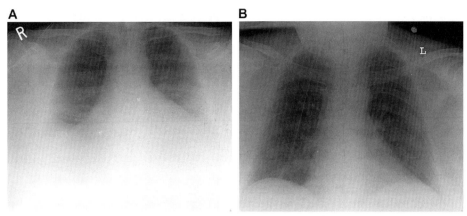

*Fig. 14.* Chest radiographs in a 57-year-old 490-lb patient. (*A*) An image of limited diagnostic quality with poor X-ray penetration and poor visualization of the lung bases. (*B*) Chest radiograph in the same patient after placement of a grid and increases in kVp and mAs. There is improved visualization of the lung bases. (*From* Uppot RN, Sahani DV, Hahn PF, et al. Impact of obesity on medical imaging and image-guided intervention. AJR Am J Roentgenol 2007;188(2):436; with permission from the American Journal of Roentgenology.)

inincreased noise, decreased image contrast, geometric unsharpness, and greater potential for motion unsharpness. [33]. Increased adipose tissue also has been correlated with increased rates of recall and false-positive screening mammograms [8,9].

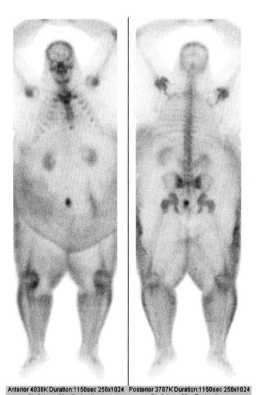

Anterior 4038K Duration:1150sec 256x1024    Posterior 3787K Duration:1150sec 256x1024
Pix:2.4mm 99m Technetium                    Pix:2.4mm 99m Technetium

*Fig. 15.* Technetium-99m bone scan in a 60-year-old man to look for osteomyelitis. Photon scatter and soft tissue attenuation limit the image quality. (*From* Uppot RN, Sahani DV, Hahn PF, et al. Impact of obesity on medical imaging and image-guided intervention. AJR Am J Roentgenol 2007;188(2):440; with permission from the American Journal of Roentgenology.)

## Nuclear medicine and positron emission tomography CT

Nuclear medicine studies can be compromised by obesity. Obesity impacts nuclear medicine in terms of table weight limits and limitations in the dose of radioisotopes that can be administered.

### Table weight

Bone scans performed with dual-head cameras are limited to the 400-lb weight limit of the table. Not all nuclear medicine studies need to be performed on the study tables, however. Many gamma cameras are portable and can be wheeled to the patient's stretcher to perform the study.

### Radioisotope factors

Administered radioisotopes may be degraded by the scatter of photons within the soft tissues, which can decrease the signal-to-noise ratio [21] (Fig. 15). Also, because the administration of radioisotopes is based on weight (mCi/kg), obese patients may exceed the maximum allowable dose and may not be able to receive the proportionate dose of the radioisotope for their body weight, further decreasing the signal-to-noise ratio. Solutions to these problems include using the maximum allowable radioisotope dose, using the highest field gamma cameras, and imaging the patient for longer time periods to maximize counts.

## Interventional radiology

Interventional radiology in obese patients can be a challenge. In addition to the imaging limitations for CT, ultrasound, and fluoroscopy, discussed previously, limitations include instrument length, the ability to fit both the patient and the instruments into the bore/gantry, patient positioning for the procedure, the ability to sedate the patient safely, and higher risks for postprocedure complications.

### Instrument length

All wires and catheters used for interventional radiology are designed with specific lengths. The longest standard instrument lengths are as follows: coaxial introducer/vascular access needles, 15 cm; biopsy needle, 25 cm; sheaths, 25 cm; dilators, 20 cm; drainage catheters, 25 cm; and RF probes, 25 cm. The challenge in obese patients comes when the thickness of the subcutaneous fat approaches the length of the instruments. Thick, soft tissues also can limit the ability to palpate or ultrasound the vessels. A recent abstract presented at the 2005 annual meeting of the Radiologic Society of North America discussed how the length of injection needles for administering medication via the buttocks is not long enough to reach the gluteal muscles in obese patients because of the thickness of the gluteal fat [34].

### Solutions for improved interventional access in obese patients

Preplanning is required to estimate lengths and distances accurately. This process can be accomplished by reviewing prior imaging studies and positioning the patient properly to access the vessel, lesion, or collection in the shortest possible distance. In addition, landmarks can be used to estimate the trajectory path to the vessel, lesion, or collection. Furthermore, it is important to understand that the soft tissues have approximately 1 to 2 cm of pliability. A distance 1 to 2 cm longer than the length of a given instrument may be reachable by pushing down on and displacing the soft tissues (Fig. 16).

### Ability to fit both the patient and instruments into the bore/gantry

A limitation commonly seen with CT-guided procedures is inadequate clearance space for the patient and the instrument into the gantry. Several solutions exist for this problem, including proper patient positioning allowing for the shortest distance to the lesion or collection with the largest clearance space, the use of real-time CT fluoroscopy to advance the instruments using a different angle, and the use of a tandem approach in which a shorter needle is inserted and its trajectory is used to place

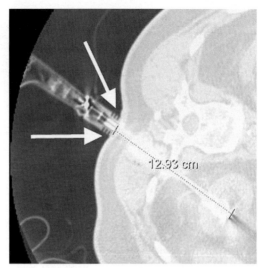

*Fig. 16.* Axial CT in a radiofrequency ablation procedure shows pliability of the subcutaneous fat that allows the probe to be pushed in further to gain a length advantage (*arrows*).

the longer needle. Also, many manufacturers of RF and cryoablation probes are addressing this issue of clearance by designing probes that have right-angle handles (to allow the handles of the instrument to clear the gantry) or that are flexible (so that they can be bent to clear the gantry for imaging) (Fig. 17). Manufacturers of larger-bore CT scanners also have begun to market their equipment for interventional procedures.

### Patient positioning

Proper patient positioning is important for image-guided procedures in obese patients. Gantry clearance and the shortest distance to the pathology are important considerations. Although pillows and splints for patient positioning exist, sandbags and other devices typically reserved for use in the operating room may be used to position a patient properly. These devices allow the patient to remain securely positioned for the duration of the procedure.

### Patient sedation

Properly sedating an obese patient for an image-guided procedure requires addressing airway management and adequacy of pain control. Airway management is an important issue to address before conscious sedation in an obese patient. Many obese patients have increased neck soft tissue and obstructive sleep apnea. Simple conscious sedation in this group of patients with midazolam hydrochloride and sublimaze fentanyl may cause airway

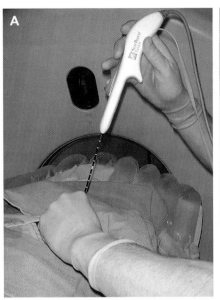
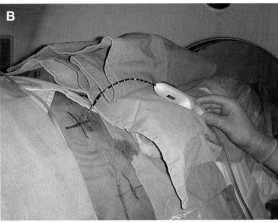

*Fig. 17.* Radiofrequency ablation procedure. (*A*) Insertion of radiofrequency probe into the liver. Note minimal clearance space for the probe and the obese patient into the CT gantry. (*B*) The radiofrequency probe is flexible and can bend, allowing the probe to clear the gantry for imaging.

compromise. In such cases, an anesthesia consultation may be required for proper airway control.

Pain control may be difficult in obese patients because of the larger sedative doses required. Local anesthetics such as lidocaine have a maximum limit of 300 mg (30 cm$^3$ of 1% lidocaine). Medications for intravenous conscious sedation are weight based (midazolam hydrochloride, 0.01–0.05 mg/kg; sublimaze fentanyl, 0.5–3 µg/kg) but do not have an absolute maximum dose as long as cardiac and respiratory functions are monitored closely. Even high doses may not be adequate to control pain in obese patients, however, and consideration must given to using a different mixture of medications (ie, meperidine and morphine) or general anesthesia.

### Postprocedure complications

As with any surgical procedure, obese patients are at increased risk for wound infections and wound breakdown because of the increased associated comorbidities such as diabetes and heart disease. In addition, the soft tissue bulk may strain healing wounds. Also, postprocedure pain in obese patients may not be controlled adequately with standard narcotics, and patient-controlled analgesia pumps may be required.

### Summary

With the increasing prevalence of obesity in the United States and around the world, the impact of this condition will become more profound.

Increasingly, obesity is becoming an issue for radiologists and radiology departments. Radiologists must be cognizant of the limitations of their imaging equipment and must be able to make the necessary technical and equipment adjustments to obtain quality imaging in obese patients. Advances in CT and MR imaging equipment with larger apertures and larger table weight limits are addressing the problems of equipment design. Technological advances including harmonics in ultrasound, dual-source CT, and increased gradient strengths and matrix coils in MR imaging are poised to address the issues of limited image quality in obese patients.

### References

[1] Uppot RN, Sahani DV, Hahn PF, et al. Effect of obesity on image quality: fifteen-year longitudinal study for evaluation of dictated radiology reports. Radiology 2006;240:435–9.

[2] Centers for Disease Control and Prevention. Overweight and obesity: obesity trends—1991–2001. Prevalence of obesity among U.S. adults by state. Available at: http://www.cdc.gov/nccdphp/dnpa/obesity/consequences.htm. Accessed April 6, 2007.

[3] Rundle RL. U.S.'s obesity woes put a strain on hospitals in unexpected ways. Wall Street Journal online edition. May 1, 2002. Available at: online.wsj.com/article/0,SB1020194636122710680.djm,00.html. Accessed September 1, 2006.

[4] Diconsiglio J. Hospitals equip to meet the bariatric challenge. Rising number of obese patients

necessitates specific supplies. Mater Manag Health Care 2006;15(4):36–9.

[5] National Task Force on the Prevention and Treatment of Obesity. Medical care for obese patients: advice for health care professionals. Am Fam Physician 2002;65(1):81–8.

[6] Padilla LA, Radosevich DM, Milad MP. Limitations of the pelvic examination for evaluation of the female pelvic organs. Int J Gynaecol Obstet 2005;88(1):84–8.

[7] Wittmer MH, Duszak R, Lewis ER, et al. Does obesity degrade image quality of helical CT for suspected pulmonary embolism? Abstracts of the 104th Annual Roentgen Ray Society Meeting. Miami Beach (FL), 2004. p. 113.

[8] Elmore JG, Carney PA, Abraham LA, et al. The association between obesity and screening mammography accuracy. Arch Intern Med 2004; 164(10):1140–7.

[9] Hunt KA, Sickles EA. Effect of obesity on screening mammography: outcomes analysis of 88,346 consecutive examinations. AJR Am J Roentgenol 2000;174:1251–5.

[10] Halpern BS, Dahlbom M, Quon A, et al. Impact of patient weight and emission scan duration on PET/CT image quality and lesion detectability. J Nucl Med 2004;45(5):797–801.

[11] Inge TH, Donnelly LF, Vierra M, et al. Managing bariatric patients in a children's hospital: radiologic considerations and limitations. J Pediatr Surg 2005;40(4):609–17.

[12] Cheadle WG. Risk factors for surgical site infection. Surg Infect (Larchmt) 2006;7(Suppl 1):S7–11.

[13] Ogan OU, Plevak DJ. Anesthetic safety always an issue with obstructive sleep apnea. J Clin Monit Comput 1998;14(1):69–70.

[14] Parlow JL, Ahn R, Milne B. Obesity is a risk factor for failure of "fast track" extubation following coronary artery bypass surgery. Can J Anaesth 2006;53(3):288–94.

[15] Montgomery JS, Gayed BA, Hollenbeck BK, et al. Obesity adversely affects health related quality of life before and after radical retropubic prostatectomy. J Urol 2006;176(1):257–62.

[16] Rosenthal K. Selecting the best i.v. site for an obese patient. Nursing 2004;34(11):14.

[17] Mei Z, Grummer-Strawn LM, Pietrobelli A, et al. Validity of body mass index compared with other body-composition screening indexes for the assessment of body fatness in children and adolescents. Am J Clin Nutr 2002;75(6):978–85.

[18] Garrow JS, Webster J. Quetelet's index (W/H2) as a measure of fatness. Int J Obes 1985;9:147–53.

[19] Nevill AM, Stewart AD, Olds T, et al. Relationship between adiposity and body size reveals limitations of BMI. Am J Phys Anthropol 2006; 129(1):151–6.

[20] Romero-Corral A, Montori VM, Somers VK, et al. Association of bodyweight with total mortality and with cardiovascular events in coronary artery disease: a systematic review of cohort studies. Lancet 2006;368(9536):666–78.

[21] Uppot RN, Sahani DV, Hahn PF, et al. Impact of obesity on medical imaging and image-guided intervention. AJR Am J Roentgenol 2007;188(2): 433–40.

[22] Statistics related to overweight and obesity. A U.S weight control information network. Available at: http://win.niddk.nih.gov/statistics/#preval. Accessed September 12, 2005.

[23] Dallessio KM. Multislice CT for imaging morbidly obese patients. Appl Radiol 2005;34(10): 38–9.

[24] Gastric bypass surgery popularity leads to jump in plastic surgery procedures, according to ASPS statistics. Available at: http://www.plasticsurgery.org/media/press_releases/Gastric-Bypass-Surgery-Popularity-Leads-to-Jump-in-Plastic-Surgery-Procedures.cfm. Accessed April 6, 2006.

[25] Trus TL, Pope GD, Finlayson SR. National trends in utilization and outcomes of bariatric surgery. Surg Endosc 2005;19(5):616–20.

[26] Kumar S, Moro L, Narayan Y. Perceived physical stress at work and musculoskeletal discomfort in X-ray technologists. Ergonomics 2004;47(2): 189–201.

[27] Shapiro RS, Wagreich J, Parsons RB, et al. Tissue harmonic imaging sonography: evaluation of image quality compared with conventional sonography. AJR Am J Roentgenol 1998;171: 1203–6.

[28] Hann LE, Bach AM, Cramer LD, et al. Hepatic sonography: comparison of tissue harmonic and standard sonography techniques. AJR Am J Roentgenol 1999;173:201–6.

[29] Vannier MW. MDCT of massively obese patients n Stanford radiology. Presented at the 8th Annual International Symposium on Multidetector-Row CT. Stanford (CA), June 14–17, 2006.

[30] Vannier MW, Johnson PJ, Dachman A, et al. Multidetector CT of massively obese patients. Presented at the 2005 meeting of the Radiological Society of North America (RSNA). Chicago (IL), November 27–December 12, 2005.

[31] Kalra M, Schmidt B, Suess C, et al. Comparison of single and dual source 64 channel MDCT scanner for evaluation of large patients: a phantom study. Presented at the 2005 meeting of the Radiological Society of North America (RSNA). Chicago (IL), November 27–December 12, 2005.

[32] Uppot RN, Sheehan A, Seethamraju R. MRI hot topic obesity and MR imaging. Malvern (PA): Siemens Medical Solutions; 2005.

[33] Guest AR, Helvie MA, Chan HP, et al. Adverse effects of increased body weight on quantitative measures of mammographic image quality. AJR Am J Roentgenol 2000;175:805–10.

[34] Chan V, Colville J, Persaud T, et al. Intramuscular injections into the buttocks: are they truly intramuscular? Presented at the 2005 meeting of the Radiological Society of North America (RSNA). Chicago (IL), November 27–December 12, 2005.

ELSEVIER
SAUNDERS

RADIOLOGIC
CLINICS
OF NORTH AMERICA

Radiol Clin N Am 45 (2007) 247–260

# Imaging Evaluation Following Roux-en-Y Gastric Bypass Surgery for Morbid Obesity

Laura R. Carucci, MD*, Mary Ann Turner, MD, Jinxing Yu, MD

Morbid obesity has become a major health problem in Western countries and continues to increase in epidemic proportions [1,2]. There has been a reported 74% increase in the prevalence of obesity from 1991 to 2001 in the United States alone, and currently more than 50% of adults are considered overweight or obese as defined by a body mass index greater than 25 kg/m² [1,3–7]. Obesity places a tremendous burden on health care because of the associated disability, comorbidities, and early mortality [1–3,5,8–13].

Because nonsurgical approaches to weight loss have limited long-term efficacy for the treatment of morbid obesity, bariatric surgery is on the rise [1,11,14,15]. Bariatric surgery has been shown to be a more effective treatment for morbid obesity in terms of decreased morbidity, sustained weight loss, reversal of comorbidities, and prolonged life expectancy [1,4,11,16–18]. As a consequence, bariatric surgery has become a common procedure performed in both large academic centers and in the private practice setting. The highest long term success rates for bariatric surgery have been reported with the Roux-en-Y gastric bypass procedure (RYGBP), and the RYGBP is considered by many in the United States to be the bariatric procedure of choice [1,10,11,14,15,18–25].

Despite the success of RYGBP, many complications may occur. After RYGBP, patients frequently are evaluated with postoperative upper gastrointestinal (UGI) examinations and CT, and it is important for radiologists to be aware of the expected postoperative findings and the potential complications that may occur in the early postoperative setting and with long-term follow-up.

---

Department of Radiology, Abdominal Imaging Section, Virginia Commonwealth University Medical Center, 1250 East Marshall St., Main Hospital 3rd Floor, Room 3-417, P.O. Box 980615, Richmond, VA 23298-0615, USA
* Corresponding author.
*E-mail address:* lcarucci@vcu.edu (L.R. Carucci).

doi:10.1016/j.rcl.2007.03.006

## Roux-en-Y gastric bypass procedure

The RYGBP may be performed with either a laparoscopic or open surgical approach. With either technique, a small gastric fundal pouch is created to exclude the remainder of the stomach, duodenum, and proximal jejunum from the path of food. The small gastric pouch is anastomosed to a jejunal Roux-limb by a narrow gastrojejunal stoma that typically is 8 to 15 mm in diameter. This procedure creates a short blind-ending jejunal limb and an antegrade-flowing jejunal limb. There is subsequently a distal side-to-side jejuno-jejunal anastomosis between the antegrade-flowing jejunal limb and the excluded jejunal limb (Fig. 1A). Ingested contents are expected to course from the esophagus into the small gastric pouch, through the narrow gastrojejunal anastomosis, into the antegrade-flowing jejunal limb, and subsequently into the distal small bowel. This procedure results in weight loss because of early satiety from the small gastric pouch and narrow gastrojejunal stoma as well as decreased absorption resulting from bypassing the proximal jejunum [1,23,26].

## Technique and expected imaging findings after Roux-en-Y gastric bypass procedure: upper gastrointestinal examination and CT

UGI and small bowel follow-through (SBFT) examinations may be performed in the early postoperative setting to assess for postoperative complications including leak, postoperative edema, ileus, and obstruction. Radiologic evaluation is important to aid in the diagnosis of early postoperative complications, because clinical evaluation may be difficult in this patient population. In addition, gastric pouch and gastrojejunal stomal size may be assessed.

In the early postoperative period, patients are evaluated initially using water-soluble contrast material. After a preliminary overhead radiograph, the patient is placed in the supine left posterior oblique position, and contrast material is administered. Adequate distention of the gastric pouch and gastrojejunal anastomosis is essential to assess accurately for postoperative leak. The supine position is preferred over the upright position: postoperative leaks may be missed if the patient is evaluated only in the upright position, due to inadequate distention of the gastric pouch. Also, the supine position allows an immediate postoperative UGI examination as indicated.

Special attention is initially directed to the postsurgical area in the left upper quadrant of the abdomen. Fluoroscopically, contrast material is observed to flow from the esophagus into the small gastric pouch, through the gastrojejunal anastomosis, and into the two jejunal limbs (Fig. 1B). Fluoroscopic images are acquired, documenting the distal esophagus, gastric pouch, gastrojejunal anastomosis, and proximal jejunum. The authors have found that the left posterior oblique position allows the most optimal assessment of the proximal anastomosis in the majority of the patients. Additional fluoroscopic views are obtained as indicated. Once no leak has been identified with water-soluble

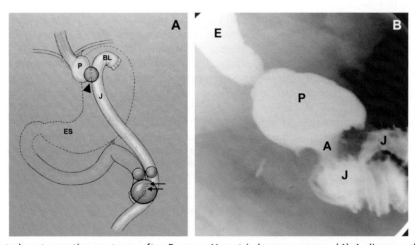

**Fig. 1.** Expected postoperative anatomy after Roux-en-Y gastric bypass surgery. (*A*) A diagram depicting the surgical procedure shows a small gastric pouch (*P*) with an anastomosis (*arrowhead*) to a Roux jejunal limb. This procedure creates a blind-ending jejunal limb (*BL*) and an antegrade-flowing jejunal limb (*J*) with a distal side-to-side jejuno-jejunal anastomosis (*arrows*). The remainder of the stomach is excluded from the path of food (*ES*). (*B*) Fluoroscopic spot image from an UGI examination with the patient in the left posterior oblique position shows the distal esophagus (*E*), gastric pouch (*P*), gastrojejunal anastomosis (*A*) and two jejunal limbs (*J*).

contrast material, barium is administered. Overhead radiographs are obtained at 20- to 30-minute intervals after the fluoroscopic examination until contrast passes distal to the distal small bowel anastomosis. It is important to ensure that contrast material has passed the distal small bowel anastomosis, because leak and/or obstruction may occur at this site as well.

In the delayed postoperative setting, patients may be evaluated for failed weight loss or weight gain, nonspecific abdominal pain, obstruction, and internal or ventral hernia. Oral barium is administered, and the examination again is performed initially in the supine left posterior oblique position with attention directed toward the proximal anastomosis. Once adequate fluoroscopic images of the postoperative anatomy have been obtained, the proximal and mid esophagus may be assessed. Contrast material then is followed to the level of the terminal ileum, because complications, including small bowel obstruction, ventral hernia, adhesions,

and internal hernia, may not become apparent until the small bowel is completely opacified with contrast material. The small bowel, including the terminal ileum, is evaluated fluoroscopically, and the anterior abdominal wall is evaluated for ventral hernia with the patient performing a Valsalva's maneuver in the straight lateral position.

Radiologists also must be aware of the typical postoperative appearance on CT after RYGBP (Fig. 2). CT examinations ideally are performed with both oral and intravenous contrast. Technical factors may have to be altered because of increased patient size; increases in kVp and mAs and thicker collimation may be necessary. Knowledge of the postoperative anatomy ensures proper identification of the excluded gastric fundus rather than the misdiagnosis of a left upper quadrant abscess. In addition, because of the altered postoperative configuration of small bowel, complications such as small bowel obstruction may produce varying patterns, as discussed later.

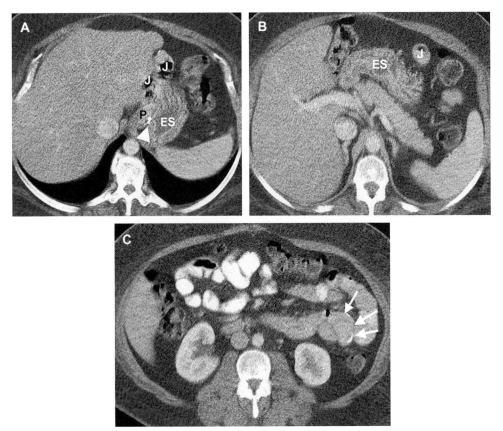

*Fig. 2.* Expected postoperative anatomy on CT after RYGBP. (*A*) Axial contrast-enhanced CT image shows the expected postoperative anatomy including the gastric pouch (*P*), the gastric staple line (*arrowhead*), the two jejunal limbs (*J*), and the excluded stomach (*ES*). (*B*) Axial contrast-enhanced CT image slightly more caudally shows the decompressed, unopacified excluded stomach (*ES*). The Roux jejunal limb (*J*) is anterior and to the left of the excluded stomach (*ES*) (*C*) Axial contrast-enhanced CT image through the mid abdomen shows the distal jejuno-jejunal anastomosis (*arrows*).

## Complications after Roux-en-Y gastric bypass procedure

Although RYGBP surgery has been shown to have a high success rate in terms of sustained weight loss and decreased obesity-related comorbidities, many complications may occur. Box 1 depicts complications that may occur in the early period (within 1 month after surgery) and in the late postoperative time course.

### Postoperative leak

Postoperative extraluminal leak is the most common serious complication after RYGBP, and leaks may occur in up to 6% of patients [1,5,19,24,27–30]. If not recognized early and treated promptly, postoperative leak is a potentially lethal complication of bariatric surgery [23,28,30,31]. Extraluminal leak requires repeat surgery in up to 80% of patients [30]. In addition, postoperative leak prolongs the hospital course and increases the morbidity and mortality after RYGBP [27,30–33].

Radiologic contrast studies often are essential to aid in the diagnosis of postoperative leak, because clinical findings may be nonspecific, and physical examination may be difficult because of patient size [26,31,33]. Postoperative leak is diagnosed most often within 10 days after surgery, and routine planned, early postoperative UGI examinations may minimize the morbidity associated with postoperative leak. [30,31,34].

Seventy-seven percent of postoperative leaks after RYGBP occur at the gastrojejunal anastomosis (Fig. 3) [30]. Leak also may arise from the distal esophagus, gastric pouch, blind-ending jejunal limb (Fig. 4), or, rarely, from the jejuno-jejunal anastomosis [30]. Up to 75% of postoperative leaks result in left upper quadrant fluid collections that

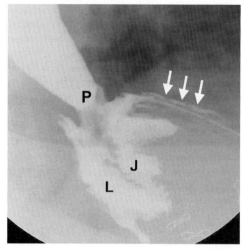

*Fig. 3.* Postoperative leak from the gastrojejunal anastomosis. A fluoroscopic UGI image in the left posterior oblique position shows a leak from the gastrojejunal anastomosis extending both to the left and right of the anastomosis with a small collection of extraluminal contrast material (*L*) and leakage of contrast material to opacify a surgical drain (*arrows*). J, jejunum; P, pouch.

can be seen on UGI examination or CT (see Fig. 4; Fig. 5) [30]. It is important to assess carefully for contrast material entering a surgical drain (see Fig. 3), because this may be the only indication of

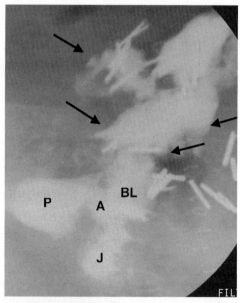

*Fig. 4.* Postoperative leak from the blind-ending jejunal limb. A fluoroscopic UGI image in the left posterior oblique position shows a leak from the blind-ending jejunal limb (*BL*) with a large extraluminal collection of contrast material extending into the left upper quadrant (*arrows*). A, gastrojejunal anastomosis; J, jejunum; P, pouch.

---

### Box 1: Complications after Roux-en-Y gastric bypass procedure

*Early*
Postoperative leak
Stomal edema/hematoma
Ileus
Obstruction
Distended excluded stomach
Staple-line disruption

*Late*
Staple-line disruption
Stomal stenosis
Obstruction
Internal hernia
Abdominal wall hernia
Marginal ulcer

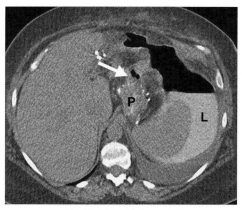

*Fig. 5.* Postoperative leak with a left upper quadrant fluid collection. Axial CT image shows the gastric pouch (*P*) and a large subphrenic and perisplenic collection of extraluminal gas and contrast material (*L*) caused by leak from the gastrojejunal anastomosis (*arrow*).

leak and may be seen best on follow-up overhead radiographs. Postoperative leak may result in peritonitis, abscesses (most often left subphrenic in location), and chronic fistulae [26,28,30,31].

*Potential pitfalls that may mimic extraluminal leak on upper gastrointestinal examination*
Experience with UGI studies after RYGBP is important, because several findings may be mistaken for free leak, including postoperative plication defects, communication with the excluded stomach, and retrograde flow of contrast material into the excluded stomach.

Postoperative plication defects are focal areas of out-pouching and deformity along the gastric pouch or extending along the gastrojejunal anastomosis itself (Fig. 6). These defects typically are associated with suture lines. Contrast material within

a focal out-pouching could be mistaken for free leak. A plication defect, however, readily fills and empties with contrast material during the fluoroscopic examination and has well-defined margins. In addition, larger plication defects may demonstrate normal gastric rugal folds. Proper technique with adequate distention of the gastric pouch usually show the true nature of the finding.

A leakage of contrast material across the gastric staple line into the excluded stomach may be mistaken for free leak as well. This differentiation is important, because communication with the excluded stomach does not have the associated increased morbidity and mortality of free leak. In this setting, contrast material is contained within the bowel. On fluoroscopic examination, a small collection of contrast material may extend to the left of the gastrojejunal anastomosis. However, normal gastric rugal folds can be identified within this collection (Fig. 7A). In addition, when the patient is repositioned right-side-down at fluoroscopy, contrast material can be seen to enter the more distal excluded stomach and duodenum (Fig. 7B). These observations confirm an intragastric location of contrast material.

Contrast material also may enter the excluded stomach by retrograde flow into the excluded limb. This occurrence happens most often in the setting of ileus or downstream obstruction. On follow-up overhead radiographs, this occurrence also can result in contrast material in the left upper quadrant in the vicinity of the gastrojejunal anastomosis (Fig. 8). This situation can be differentiated from free leak because this is a delayed finding that is revealed only on follow-up overhead radiographs and is not seen on initial fluoroscopic examination. Contrast material often is also present in the duodenum and excluded limb (see Fig. 8).

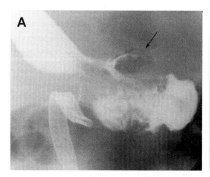
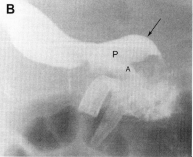

*Fig. 6.* Postoperative plication defect: a pitfall that may mimic free leak. (*A, B*). Serial UGI fluoroscopic spot images in the left posterior oblique position show a large plication defect along the lateral aspect of the gastric pouch (*P in panel B*) apposing the gastrojejunal anastomosis (*A in panel B*). (*A*) The initial spot image shows a linear collection of contrast material and gas extending laterally from the anastomosis (*arrow*). (*B*) Adequate distention shows that this contrast material is in a large area of postoperative deformity (a plication defect) along the gastric pouch (*arrow*) rather than a leak.

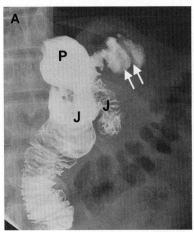
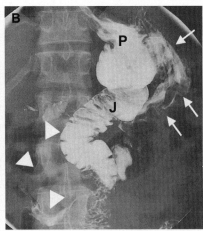

*Fig. 7.* Leakage of contrast material across the gastric staple line into the excluded stomach (staple-line disruption): a pitfall that may mimic free leak. (*A*) A fluoroscopic UGI spot image shows a small collection of contrast material to the left of the gastrojejunal anastomosis that could be mistaken for free leak. Gastric rugal folds (*arrows*) can be identified within the collection, however, a finding consistent with leak into the excluded stomach rather than free leak. There is preferential flow into jejunum (*J*). P, gastric pouch. (*B*) After the patient is rotated to the right, a small amount of contrast material is seen opacifying the excluded stomach (*arrows*) and the excluded duodenum (*arrowheads*). J, jejunum; P, gastric pouch.

### Early postoperative obstruction

With routine early postoperative UGI examinations, an adynamic ileus is a common finding. It is important to differentiate early postoperative obstruction from ileus. Early postoperative

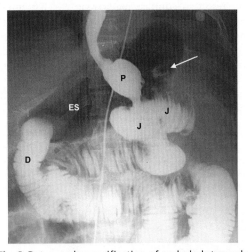

*Fig. 8.* Retrograde opacification of excluded stomach: a pitfall that may mimic free leak. An overhead radiograph from an UGI examination shows a small amount of contrast material in the left upper quadrant (*arrow*) adjacent to the gastrojejunal anastomosis. There also is contrast in the excluded duodenum (*D*) from retrograde flow in the excluded limb, and there is distension of the excluded stomach (*ES*). The gastric pouch (*P*) and jejunal limbs (*J*) also are mildly dilated because of a postoperative ileus. No leak was seen at fluoroscopy.

obstruction typically is caused by edema and/or hematoma, most often involving the proximal or distal anastomosis (Figs. 9 and 10). In addition, in the setting of a retrocolic gastrojejunal anastomosis, there is often edema and/or hematoma at the site where the Roux jejunal limb crosses the transverse mesocolon (Fig. 11). Narrowing in any of these locations may produce a postoperative obstruction ranging from mild to severe. This occurrence may result in a delayed initiation of diet and a prolonged hospital course. In addition, nasogastric decompression and/or surgical intervention may be required.

A particularly important consequence of early postoperative obstruction is acute distention of the excluded stomach. If there is a downstream obstruction with acute distention of the excluded stomach, natural decompression of the excluded stomach is not possible. Overdistension of the excluded stomach may result in gastric perforation or leak from the gastrojejunal anastomosis if not treated promptly. In this setting, percutaneous needle decompression or gastrostomy catheter placement in the excluded stomach may be beneficial.

### Gastric staple-line dehiscence or disruption

A leak across the gastric staple line into the excluded stomach (gastric staple-line dehiscence or disruption) may occur in the early or late postoperative period. This occurrence allows communication between the small surgically created gastric pouch and the excluded stomach. Early disruption of the staple line may result from inadequate division of the

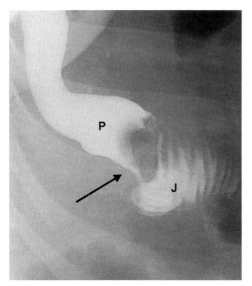

Fig. 9. Postoperative edema at the gastrojejunal anastomosis. A left posterior oblique fluoroscopic UGI image performed on postoperative day 1 shows mild dilatation of the gastric pouch (*P*) with a markedly narrowed stoma (*arrow*) caused by edema. Edema also is noted along the inferior aspect of the gastric pouch. J, jejunum.

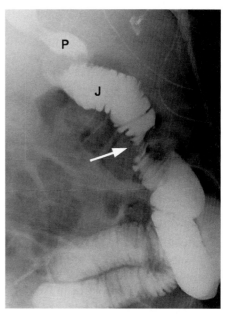

Fig. 11. Postoperative edema at the transverse mesocolic defect. An overhead radiograph from an UGI examination shows narrowing and edema where the Roux jejunal limb crosses the transverse mesocolon (*arrow*). There is mild dilatation of the proximal jejunum (*J*). P, gastric pouch.

gastric pouch at surgery. Alternatively, it may occur as a consequence of free leak [31]. Staple-line dehiscence in the late postoperative course, however, is thought to result from extensive stretching or overdistension of the gastric pouch with food [26,27,31].

Partial or complete dehiscence of the gastric staple line may result in inadequate weight loss and subsequent failed RYGBP surgery with a suboptimal clinical outcome [31,32]. Staple-line dehiscence has been reported to occur in up to 3% of patients; however, the incidence varies with the surgical technique used for the procedure [22,27]. Complete transection of the stomach at RYGBP minimizes the incidence of staple-line dehiscence.

Staple-line disruption with leak into the excluded stomach has a similar appearance at UGI examination in both the early and late postoperative course. At fluoroscopy, the excluded stomach becomes opacified as contrast exits the gastric pouch (see Fig. 7). Depending upon the degree of staple-line dehiscence, contrast may preferentially enter the excluded stomach with minimal or no opacification of the jejunal limbs, or there may be preferential flow through the gastrojejunal anastomosis into the jejunum with only a small collection of contrast material in the left upper quadrant in the excluded stomach (see Fig. 7A). An intragastric location can be confirmed by rotating the patient to the right to opacify the distal excluded stomach and duodenum (see Fig. 7B). It is important to diagnose staple-line dehiscence on the initial fluoroscopic examination because contrast material may enter

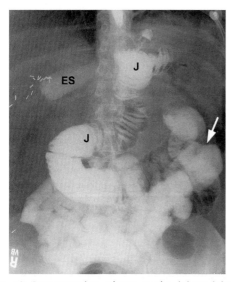

Fig. 10. Postoperative edema at the jejuno-jejunal anastomosis with mild, partial small bowel obstruction. An overhead radiograph from an UGI examination shows a dilated Roux jejunal limb (*J*) extending to the distal small bowel anastomosis (*arrow*). There also is retrograde flow into the excluded limb to opacify the excluded stomach (*ES*). Distal small bowel is decompressed.

the excluded stomach by retrograde flow on delayed overhead radiographs.

CT after RYGBP may show contrast material in the excluded stomach [35]. With CT, however, it may be difficult to assess whether contrast material entered the excluded stomach through leakage across the gastric staple line or by retrograde flow into the excluded limb. On CT, the presence of contrast material within the excluded gastric fundus without opacification of the more distal excluded stomach and duodenum may suggest leakage across the gastric staple-line (staple-line disruption). The diagnosis of staple-line disruption can be confirmed with an UGI examination.

## Stomal stenosis

Stomal or anastomotic stenosis is caused by fibrosis at the anastomosis and usually occurs 1 or more months after RYGBP, with a mean of postoperative day 49 [31,36,37]. Stomal stenosis is much more likely to occur at the gastrojejunal anastomosis than at the jejuno-jejunal anastomosis.

Stenosis at the gastrojejunal anastomosis has been reported to occur with an incidence of up to 10% of patients and is thought to be related to

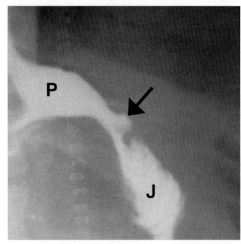

*Fig. 13.* Marginal ulcer. A fluoroscopic UGI spot image in the left posterior oblique position shows a small collection of contrast material (*arrow*) located along the gastrojejunal anastomosis consistent with a small ulcer. J, jejunum; P, pouch.

ischemic change after surgery [1,22,24,31,36–38]. Patients may present with nausea, vomiting, and excessive weight loss. On UGI examination, the esophagus and gastric pouch are dilated with delayed emptying. Often there is associated esophageal dysmotility. Depending on the degree of stenosis, the gastric pouch may have a round appearance and may contain a large amount of debris [26,31]. Dilatation of the gastric pouch may obscure the narrowed stoma on UGI examination. Gastrojejunal stomal stenosis can be treated with endoscopic dilatation, which has a success rate of up to 95% [38].

Stenosis at the jejuno-jejunal anastomosis is rare, with a reported incidence of 0.9% [31,37]. On UGI examination, partial or complete obstruction may be seen at the distal small bowel anastomosis (Fig. 12). Whereas gastrojejunal stomal stenosis typically responds well to treatment with endoscopic dilatation, stenosis at the distal anastomosis often requires surgical revision, especially if the anastomosis cannot be reached endoscopically [26].

## Marginal ulcers

After RYGBP, marginal ulcers may occur in up to 3% of patients. Marginal ulcers occur in the vicinity of the gastrojejunal anastomosis and most often occur in the jejunum adjacent to the anastomosis [22,23]. At UGI examination, a marginal ulcer appears as a small focal out-pouching of contrast material at or adjacent to the gastrojejunal anastomosis (Fig. 13). There is stasis of contrast material within the ulcer crater, often with associated adjacent fold thickening and edema. Marginal ulcers are thought

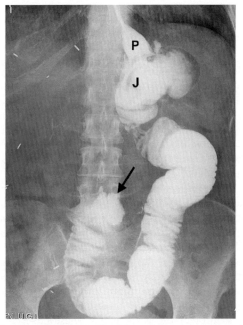

*Fig. 12.* Stenosis at the jejuno-jejunal anastomosis with small bowel obstruction. Overhead radiograph from an UGI examination in a patient 3 months after RYGBP shows dilatation of the gastric pouch (*P*) and the jejunal Roux limb (*J*) with a focal, abrupt, transition point at the distal small bowel anastomosis (*arrow*) caused by stomal stenosis. Distal bowel and bowel in the excluded limb are decompressed and are not opacified with contrast material.

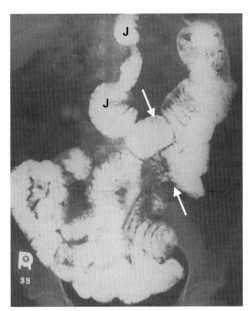

Fig. 14. Internal hernia in the left upper and mid abdomen. Overhead radiograph from an UGI examination shows an abnormal course and location of clustered small bowel in the left upper and mid abdomen. Bowel can be seen entering and exiting the hernia (*arrows*). J, jejunum.

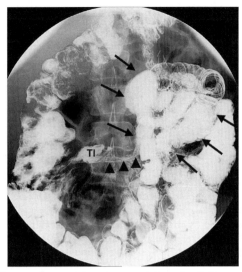

*Fig. 15.* Internal hernia containing distal ileum. A fluoroscopic spot image from an UGI examination shows an abnormal configuration of bowel with displaced and clustered distal ileum in the left upper and mid abdomen (*arrows*). The terminal ileum (*TI*) is displaced, extending from the hernia to cross the midline toward the cecum (*arrowheads*).

to occur as a consequence of exposure of the jejunal mucosa to gastric secretions and decrease in incidence with decreased gastric pouch size (smaller gastric pouches result in decreased production of gastrin and acid) [26]. Marginal ulcers usually respond well to medical management.

### Late small bowel obstruction

Small bowel obstruction may occur in up to 5% of patients in the late postoperative period after RYGBP [15,23]. Small bowel obstruction is caused most often by adhesions; other causes of obstruction after RYGBP may include internal hernia, intussusception, and abdominal wall hernias [22,23,39,40]. Obstruction also can occur at the transverse mesocolic defect (see Fig. 11). The incidence of small bowel obstruction is lower after laparoscopic surgery than after open surgery because the incidence of adhesions is lower with laparoscopic technique [22,24].

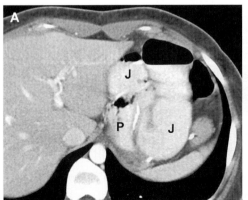
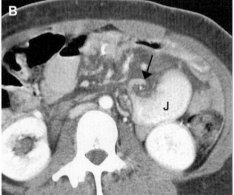

Fig. 16. Internal hernia: Petersen's hernia with volvulus. (A) Axial contrast-enhanced CT image shows dilated jejunum (J) displaced cephalad next to the gastric pouch (P). (B) Axial contrast-enhanced CT image more caudally shows dilated jejunum (J) with an abrupt transition point. There is an associated swirling appearance of mesenteric vessels (*arrow*) with engorgement of the mesentery.

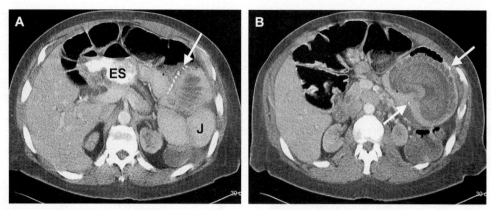

*Fig. 17.* Fixed intussusception at the jejuno-jejunal anastomosis with small bowel obstruction. (*A*) Axial contrast-enhanced CT image shows a dilated Roux jejunal limb (*J*) in the left mid abdomen. A left mid abdominal suture line for the jejuno-jejunal anastomosis (*arrow*) is noted. The excluded stomach (*ES*) is decompressed. (*B*) Axial CT image more inferiorly shows a jejuno-jejunal intussusception with the distal small bowel anastomotic suture line acting as a lead point (*arrows*). There is marked edema of the associated mesentery.

## Internal hernia

Internal hernia is a rare, potentially fatal, complication of RYGBP that has been reported in up to 3% of patients [22,24,36,39]. The development of internal hernia varies with surgical approach: there is an increased incidence of internal hernia after laparoscopic RYGBP [22,23]. Although internal hernia can occur at any time after RYGBP, it

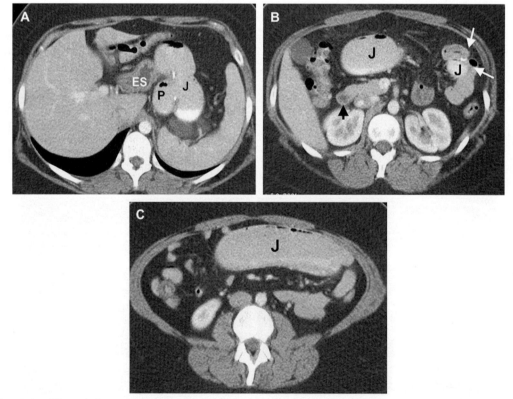

*Fig. 18.* Small bowel obstruction at the distal small bowel anastomosis: dilated Roux jejunal limb. (*A, B, C*) Axial contrast-enhanced CT images show marked dilatation of the gastric pouch (*P*) and the Roux jejunal limb (*J*) extending to the point of the distal small bowel anastomosis (*white arrows*). Distal small bowel and the excluded limb including the excluded stomach (*ES*) and duodenum (*black arrow*) are decompressed.

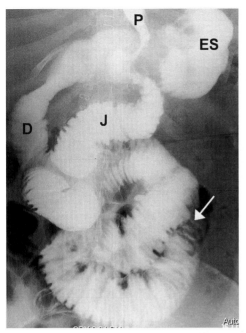

*Fig. 19.* Small bowel obstruction at the distal small bowel anastomosis: dilated Roux jejunal limb and excluded limb. Overhead radiograph from an UGI examination shows a small bowel obstruction at the jejuno-jejunal anastomosis (*arrow*) with a dilated Roux jejunal limb (*J*) and with retrograde flow into the excluded limb with opacification of the excluded stomach (*ES*) and duodenum (*D*). There is no contrast opacification of bowel distal to the small bowel anastomosis. P, gastric pouch.

typically occurs in the late postoperative course, more than 1 month after surgery [22].

Postoperative internal hernia occurs when there is a herniation of bowel through a mesenteric defect. Although internal hernia may occur through any surgically created defect, the most common sites are through the defect in the transverse mesocolon for the Roux-jejunal limb, in the region of the distal small bowel anastomosis, and posterior to the Roux limb (Petersen's defect), respectively [39]. Internal hernia may cause obstruction and may lead to volvulus, infarction, and perforation of bowel. It can be a devastating complication of RYGBP, especially if diagnosis and treatment are delayed.

The clinical presentation of internal hernia may be nonspecific with intermittent abdominal pain or a sudden onset of abdominal pain, and a high index of suspicion is required to make the diagnosis. Therefore, it is imperative for radiologists to be aware of this potential complication of RYGBP and to be familiar with the findings that may be seen at SBFT and on CT studies.

On both SBFT and CT studies, an atypical bowel configuration is noted with a clustered appearance of bowel (Figs. 14–16). Clustered loops of small bowel often displace other bowel. There may be a visible loop of small bowel entering and exiting the clustered segment (see Fig. 14). Abnormally clustered and displaced small bowel is located most often in the left abdomen (see Fig. 14) but can be seen anywhere in the abdomen and pelvis. Small bowel obstruction may or may not be present at the time of the study. On SBFT studies, there is a visible change in the configuration of bowel and/or in the location of the distal anastomotic suture line in comparison with a prior postoperative study. Small bowel loops are fixed and may remain clustered even with the patient in the upright position. There often is associated stasis within clustered small bowel loops. On CT, stretching and/or displacement of the associated mesenteric vessels with mesenteric engorgement may be identified (see Fig. 16). Adhesions also may result in a fixed and tethered appearance of small bowel, and differentiation of internal hernia from adhesions may be difficult [41].

### Incisional hernia

Ventral or incisional hernia is a common complication after open RYGBP, occurring in up to 24% of patients. Small bowel obstruction is rare after open surgery, however, because of the very large neck of a ventral hernia. Incisional hernias are much less common after laparoscopic RYGBP but may occur at laparoscopic port sites and can result in obstruction and/r strangulation of bowel because of the small size of the hernia neck [24,37].

### Intussusception

Intussusception after RYGBP is rare. It occurs most often at the jejuno-jejunal anastomosis, because the anastomotic suture line acts as a lead point. Intussusception may be a transient or fixed finding and can result in small bowel obstruction (Fig. 17) [40].

### Patterns of small bowel obstruction after Roux-en-Y gastric bypass procedure

After RYGBP, small bowel obstruction on CT or SBFT may not follow the typical pattern of obstruction expected in patients without a Roux limb. An accurate diagnosis of small bowel obstruction after RYGBP requires knowledge of the expected postoperative anatomy, and it is important to be aware of the various patterns of small bowel obstruction that may occur in relationship to the jejuno-jejunal anastomosis.

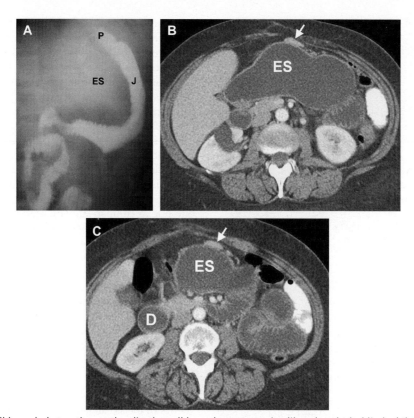

**Fig. 20.** Small bowel obstruction at the distal small bowel anastomosis: dilated excluded limb. (*A*) Overhead radiograph from an UGI examination shows contrast material opacifying the gastric pouch (*P*) and antegrade-flowing jejunal limb (*J*). The Roux limb is not dilated; however, it is compressed and displaced by the dilated, fluid-filled excluded stomach (*ES*). (*B, C*) Axial contrast-enhanced CT images show the dilated, unopacified, fluid-filled excluded limb including the excluded stomach (*ES*), duodenum (*D*), and left mid abdominal jejunum. The Roux jejunal limb is decompressed and is displaced anteriorly (*arrows*).

Small bowel obstruction can occur at the jejuno-jejunal anastomosis with dilatation of only the proximal Roux-jejunal limb. In this setting, the gastric pouch may be distended, and the antegrade-flowing jejunal limb is dilated and fluid filled leading up to the small bowel anastomosis, typically in the left mid to lower abdomen (see Fig. 12; Fig. 18). Alternatively, small bowel obstruction at the jejuno-jejunal anastomosis may occur so that the jejunal Roux limb and the excluded limb are both dilated. The excluded limb is dilated by retrograde flow. Upon imaging, there is distention of the proximal Roux jejunal limb, as well as the excluded stomach, duodenum, and jejunum, with retrograde flow into the excluded limb (Fig. 19). Small bowel distal to the small bowel anastomosis is decompressed. This pattern of obstruction exerts pressure on the excluded stomach. A third pattern of obstruction related to the jejuno-jejunal anastomosis results in dilation of only the excluded limb. This pattern of obstruction can place marked pressure on the excluded stomach and stress the gastric

staple line. The excluded limb will not be opacified with contrast material on either SBFT or CT, and the dilated, fluid-filled bowel in the excluded, unopacified limb produces mass effect on the gastric pouch and Roux jejunal limb (Fig. 20).

## Summary

Understanding the expected postoperative anatomy and examination techniques after the RYGBP surgery for morbid obesity is essential to diagnose potential complications of the procedure accurately. As morbid obesity continues to increase in epidemic proportions, bariatric surgery is becoming commonplace and may even be an incidental finding at the time of imaging for other indications. Radiologists must be familiar with the expected postoperative anatomy, potential pitfalls of diagnosis, and complications that may occur after the procedure. Clinical symptomatology is often nonspecific, and physical examination may be difficult in this patient population. Proper radiologic evaluation is imperative.

# References

[1] Fisher BL, Schauer P. Medical and surgical options in the treatment of severe obesity. Am J Surg 2002; 184:9S–16S.

[2] Allison DB, Fontaine KR, Manson JE, et al. Annual deaths attributable to obesity in the United States. JAMA 1999;282:1530–8.

[3] Must A, Spadano J, Coakley EH, et al. The disease burden associated with overweight and obesity. JAMA 1999;282:1523–9.

[4] Martin LF, White S, Lindstrom W Jr. Cost-benefit analysis for the treatment of severe obesity. World J Surg 1998;22:1008–17.

[5] Livingston EH, Ko CY. Assessing the relative contribution of individual risk factors on surgical outcome for gastric bypass surgery: a baseline probability analysis. J Surg Res 2002;105:48–52.

[6] McCann J. Obesity, cancer links prompt new recommendations. J Natl Cancer Inst 2001;93:901–2.

[7] Manson JE, Skerrett PJ, Greenland P, et al. The escalating pandemics of obesity and sedentary lifestyle. A call to action for clinicians. Arch Intern Med 2004;164:249–58.

[8] Kuczmarski RJ, Flegal KM, Campbell SM, et al. Increasing prevalence of overweight among US adults. The National Health and Nutrition Examination Surveys, 1960 to 1991. JAMA 1994;272:205–11.

[9] Mokdad AH, Serdula MK, Dietz WH, et al. The spread of the obesity epidemic in the United States, 1991–1998. JAMA 1999;282:1519–22.

[10] Talieh J, Kirgan D, Fisher BL. Gastric bypass for morbid obesity: a standard surgical technique by consensus. Obes Surg 1997;7:198–202.

[11] Gastrointestinal surgery for severe obesity: National Institutes of Health Consensus Development Conference Statement. Am J Clin Nutr 1992;55:615S–9S.

[12] Calle EE, Rodriguez C, Walker-Thurmond K, et al. Overweight, obesity, and mortality from cancer in a prospectively studied cohort of U.S. adults. N Engl J Med 2003;348:1625–38.

[13] Calle EE, Thun MJ, Petrelli JM, et al. Body-mass index and mortality in a prospective cohort of U.S. adults. N Engl J Med 1999;341:1097–105.

[14] Craig BM, Tseng DS. Cost-effectiveness of gastric bypass for severe obesity. Am J Med 2002;113:491–8.

[15] Reddy RM, Riker A, Marra D, et al. Open Roux-en-Y gastric bypass for the morbidly obese in the era of laparoscopy. Am J Surg 2002;184:611–5 [discussion: 615–6].

[16] Brolin RE. Update: NIH consensus conference. Gastrointestinal surgery for severe obesity. Nutrition 1996;12:403–4.

[17] Nguyen NT, Ho HS, Palmer LS, et al. A comparison study of laparoscopic versus open gastric bypass for morbid obesity. J Am Coll Surg 2000;191:149–55 [discussion: 155–7].

[18] Lonroth H, Dalenback J. Other laparoscopic bariatric procedures. World J Surg 1998;22:964–8.

[19] Schauer PR, Ikramuddin S, Gourash W, et al. Outcomes after laparoscopic Roux-en-Y gastric bypass for morbid obesity. Ann Surg 2000;232:515–29.

[20] Sugerman HJ, Starkey JV, Birkenhauer R. A randomized prospective trial of gastric bypass versus vertical banded gastroplasty for morbid obesity and their effects on sweets versus non-sweets eaters. Ann Surg 1987;205:613–24.

[21] Sugerman HJ. Gastric bypass surgery for severe obesity. Semin Laparosc Surg 2002;9:79–85.

[22] Higa KD, Boone KB, Ho T. Complications of the laparoscopic Roux-en-Y gastric bypass: 1,040 patients–what have we learned? Obes Surg 2000;10:509–13.

[23] Fobi MA, Lee H, Holness R, et al. Gastric bypass operation for obesity. World J Surg 1998;22:925–35.

[24] DeMaria EJ, Sugerman HJ, Kellum JM, et al. Results of 281 consecutive total laparoscopic Roux-en-Y gastric bypasses to treat morbid obesity. Ann Surg 2002;235:640–5 [discussion: 645–7].

[25] Mognol P, Chosidow D, Marmuse JP. Laparoscopic gastric bypass versus laparoscopic adjustable gastric banding in the super-obese: a comparative study of 290 patients. Obes Surg 2005;15:76–81.

[26] Goodman P, Halpert RD. Radiological evaluation of gastric stapling procedures for morbid obesity. Crit Rev Diagn Imaging 1991;32:37–67.

[27] Buckwalter JA, Herbst CA Jr. Complications of gastric bypass for morbid obesity. Am J Surg 1980;139:55–60.

[28] Buckwalter JA, Herbst CA Jr. Leaks occurring after gastric bariatric operations. Surgery 1988;103:156–60.

[29] Ganci-Cerrud G, Herrera MF. Role of radiologic contrast studies in the early postoperative period after bariatric surgery. Obes Surg 1999;9:532–4.

[30] Carucci LR, Turner MA, Conklin RC, et al. Roux-en-Y gastric bypass surgery for morbid obesity: evaluation of postoperative extraluminal leaks with upper gastrointestinal series. Radiology 2006;238:119–27.

[31] Carucci LR, Turner MA. Radiologic evaluation following Roux-en-Y gastric bypass surgery for morbid obesity. Eur J Radiol 2005;53:353–65.

[32] Koehler RE, Halverson JD. Radiographic abnormalities after gastric bypass. Am J Roentgenol 1982;138:267–70.

[33] Moffat RE, Peltier GL, Jewell WR. The radiological spectrum of gastric bypass complications. Radiology 1979;132:33–6.

[34] Serafini F, Anderson W, Ghassemi P, et al. The utility of contrast studies and drains in the management of patients after Roux-en-Y gastric bypass. Obes Surg 2002;12:34–8.

[35] Yu J, Turner MA, Cho SR, et al. Normal anatomy and complications after gastric bypass surgery: helical CT findings. Radiology 2004;231:753–60.

[36] Blachar A, Federle MP, Pealer KM, et al. Gastrointestinal complications of laparoscopic Roux-en-Y gastric bypass surgery: clinical and imaging findings. Radiology 2002;223:625–32.

[37] Blachar A, Federle MP. Gastrointestinal complications of laparoscopic roux-en-Y gastric bypass surgery in patients who are morbidly obese: findings on radiography and CT. AJR 2002;179:1437–42.

[38] Go MR, Muscarella P 2nd, Needleman BJ, et al. Endoscopic management of stomal stenosis after Roux-en-Y gastric bypass. Surg Endosc 2004;18: 56–9.

[39] Higa KD, Ho T, Boone KB. Internal hernias after laparoscopic Roux-en-Y gastric bypass: incidence, treatment and prevention. Obes Surg 2003;13:350–4.

[40] Duane TM, Wohlgemuth S, Ruffin K. Intussusception after Roux-en-Y gastric bypass. Am Surg 2000;66:82–4.

[41] Blachar A, Federle MP, Dodson SF. Internal hernia: clinical and imaging findings in 17 patients with emphasis on CT criteria. Radiology 2001; 218:68–74.

RADIOLOGIC
CLINICS
OF NORTH AMERICA

Radiol Clin N Am 45 (2007) 261–274

# Adjustable Laparoscopic Gastric Banding for Morbid Obesity: Imaging Assessment and Complications

Laura R. Carucci, MD[a],*, Mary Ann Turner, MD[a],
Richard A. Szucs, MD[a,b]

- Laparoscopic adjustable gastric banding: overview
- Advantages of laparoscopic adjustable gastric banding
- Radiologic evaluation for laparoscopic adjustable gastric banding
- Fluoroscopic band adjustment
- Complications after laparoscopic adjustable gastric banding

- *Pouch dilatation*
- *Band slippage*
- *Intragastric migration of the band*
- *Problems with the port, connecting tubing, and band*
- *Esophageal dilatation and dysphasia*
- *Additional gastric complications*
- Summary
- References

Obesity is increasing in epidemic proportions and currently is the second leading cause of preventable death in the United States [1,2]. In the United States, more than 50% of adults are overweight, and more than 20% are considered obese. Furthermore, approximately 12 million Americans are considered morbidly obese as defined by a body mass index (BMI) greater than or equal to 40 kg/m$^2$ [1,3,4]. Obesity is associated with serious medical comorbidities, and society pays a high cost for this condition in terms of health care dollars and obesity-related deaths [2,4–7].

Conservative measures to achieve weight loss, including diet, exercise, and behavioral modification, have a high failure rate in the setting of morbid obesity [1,4–8]. As a consequence, surgical approaches have been developed for patients who have failed conservative treatments. According to the criteria formulated in 1991 by the National Institutes of Health consensus development conference, bariatric surgery may be considered for patients who have a BMI of 40 kg/m$^2$ or higher or of 35 to 40 kg/m$^2$ with associated high-risk obesity-related comorbidities [5,6,9–11]. In addition, patients should have failed prior conservative methods of weight loss.

Surgery for morbid obesity incorporates restrictive and/or malabsorptive procedures for the achievement of weight loss. One of the first bariatric procedures performed was the malabsorptive

[a] Department of Radiology, Abdominal Imaging Section, Virginia Commonwealth University Medical Center, 1250 East Marshall Street, Main Hospital 3rd Floor, Room 3-417, P.O. Box 980615, Richmond, VA 23298-0615, USA
[b] Commonwealth Radiology, Bon Secours St. Mary's Hospital, 5801 Bremo Road, Richmond, VA 23226, USA
* Corresponding author.
*E-mail address:* lcarucci@vcu.edu (L.R. Carucci).

radiologic.theclinics.com

doi:10.1016/j.rcl.2007.03.003

jejunoileal bypass. This procedure subsequently was abandoned because of severe metabolic and nutritional complications [5,7,8]. In more recent years, gastric restrictive procedures including horizontal and vertical gastroplasty and vertical banded gastroplasty have increased in prevalence. Other procedures such as the combined restrictive and malabsorptive Roux-en-Y gastric bypass (RYGBP) and the malabsorptive biliopancreatic diversion (BD) with or without duodenal switch also have increased in prevalence [5,8]. The RYGBP and BD are now the most commonly performed bariatric procedures in the United States and Canada, comprising 80% to 90% of bariatric procedures [12]. However, restrictive procedures remain the most popular surgical option in European countries [12–14].

Restrictive procedures work by limiting the volume of solid food that can be consumed, but liquid and semisolid high-caloric foods may pass without the sensation of satiety [12]; therefore, patient cooperation is required to maintain a restricted diet and to avoid overfeeding [12,14]. On the other hand, combined restrictive and malabsorptive bariatric procedures, such as RYGBP, result in greater sustained weight loss with less need for patient compliance; however, these procedures are more technically demanding and have higher overall morbidity [1,7,12,15].

Technically, restrictive bariatric procedures are easier to perform and have lower complication rates than RYGBP and BD; however, restrictive procedures may not be as successful for long-term weight loss, especially in superobese patients (BMI > 50 kg/m$^2$) [2,12,14–16]. Success rates for gastric restrictive procedures are better in Europe than in the United States, possibly related to differences in diet and less severe obesity in Europe [12,17]. Indeed, patients undergoing bariatric surgery in the United States tend to have a higher BMI, with more patients in the superobese category than in European countries [12].

A restrictive gastric banding procedure was first introduced in 1983, was made adjustable in 1986, and was made available laparoscopically in the early 1990s [5,8,18–20]. Because classic bariatric procedures are associated with a high complication rate and numerous side effects, the concept of a reversible, adjustable gastric banding device has become a popular alternative to more traditional bariatric procedures [21,22].

## Laparoscopic adjustable gastric banding: overview

Laparoscopic gastric banding was introduced in the early 1990s as a potentially safe, controllable, and reversible means for weight loss in morbidly obese patients [5,12,20]. The gastric banding procedure consists of placing a silicone band around the upper stomach to create a small gastric pouch and a narrow stoma that communicates with the remainder of the stomach. Initially, gastric banding devices were not adjustable, and poor weight loss occurred if the stoma was too large. If the stoma was too small, however, dysphasia and/or obstruction occurred. Subsequently, the adjustable gastric band was developed to allow percutaneous adjustment of the banding device without the need for additional surgery [8,18]. The silicone band has an adjustable inner balloon cuff that is connected by tubing to a subcutaneous injection reservoir that typically is sutured to the anterior rectus sheath (Fig. 1A). The diameter of the band may be adjusted by injecting the port to inflate the cuff (narrowing the stoma) or by aspirating fluid from the port to deflate the cuff (widening the stoma) (Fig. 1B).

Currently, the only adjustable gastric banding device approved for use in the United States by the Food and Drug Administration (approved June, 2001) is the Lap-Band adjustable gastric banding system (INAMED Health, formerly BioEnterics Corporation, Santa Barbara, CA). Although the Lap-Band has gained popularity around the world since the early 1990s and now is the leading bariatric procedure performed internationally, the Food and Drug Administration did not approve its use in the United States until 2001 [6,23]. Lap-Band placement represents less than 10% of bariatric procedures in the United States [17].

The Lap-Band is placed around the proximal stomach and contains a 4-cm inflatable cuff. Placement of the band creates a small gastric pouch with a narrow stoma. At surgery, a transesophageal calibration balloon may be placed to calibrate pouch and stomal size [8]. The pouch volume created is typically 15 cm$^3$, and initial stomal size is approximately 12 mm in diameter [5,13]. The serosa proximal and distal to the band is sutured using nonabsorbable sutures so that anterior portion of the band is covered to prevent band slippage (see Fig. 1A) [6,8,13]. The inflatable cuff is left empty following surgery, and the stoma may be adjusted postoperatively by inflating the cuff within the band [5,8,21]. The inner balloon can be inflated to contain a maximal volume of 5 cm$^3$, and the ideal stomal size is 3 to 5 mm [21]. The Lap-Band controls obesity by means of a restrictive mechanism resulting from the small gastric pouch and narrow stoma, so that the patient experiences early satiety when the pouch is full.

The Lap-Band system is the most commonly used gastric banding device worldwide. An alternative

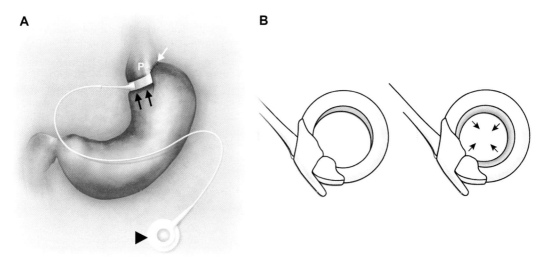

*Fig. 1.* The laparoscopic adjustable gastric band (LAGB). (*A*) The LAGB (*black arrows*) is placed around the proximal stomach to create a small gastric pouch (*P*). The band is connected to a subcutaneous reservoir (*arrowhead*) by way of connecting tubing. Note the sutures covering the band along the high greater curvature (*white arrow*). (*B*) The band device. The band is deflated on the left. On the right, arrows denote inflation of the inner cuff of the band to narrow the gastric lumen (stoma).

adjustable gastric banding device called the "Swedish adjustable gastric band" (SAGB) (ObTech Medical, 6310 Zug Switzerland) is available outside the United States. Unlike the Lap-Band, the SAGB requires injection of contrast material into the band for fluoroscopic visualization. The SAGB is a softer, wider band, and the balloon can be inflated to 9 cm$^3$. The pressure within the balloon remains low, whereas the Lap-Band is considered a high-pressure system [23]. Early band-related complications and infections may be higher with SAGB; however, long-term complication rates and weight loss rates are similar [23].

## Advantages of laparoscopic adjustable gastric banding

LAGB is the least invasive bariatric procedure, and weight loss is similar to that with other gastric restricting procedures [5,13,15,21,24,25]. The LAGB has a low complication rate and the lowest reported mortality of all bariatric procedures (<0.05%) [7,14,26]. LAGB is a reversible procedure that does not involve cutting, stapling, or bypassing portions of the gastrointestinal tract [5,8,13–15,21,23,27,28]. LAGB can adjust to the patient's situation without the need for additional surgery [25].

LAGB is technically less challenging than other procedures such as RYGBP and can be performed laparoscopically even in high-risk patients [12]. Any required reoperation usually can be performed laparoscopically with low morbidity and a short hospital stay [12,14]. In addition, if the outcome

following LAGB is suboptimal, a laparoscopic RYGBP or a combined bariatric procedure (ie, banded gastric bypass) can be performed [12,14].

Although weight loss results with LAGB may be less than with RYGBP (particularly in the superobese patient population), LAGB is safer in terms of short-term mortality and overall morbidity [1,7,15,29]. LAGB is effective in terms of weight loss with significant improvement in comorbidities [2,7,12,13,15,16,24,30,31]. Major comorbidities resolve in 50% to 80% of patients and improve in 10% to 40% of patients following LAGB [12]. Furthermore, studies show that LAGB results in improved quality of life in 82% of patients, with maximal weight loss occurring within the first 2 to 3 years following the procedure [12,14].

## Radiologic evaluation for laparoscopic adjustable gastric banding

An upper gastrointestinal (UGI) examination is helpful before LAGB to evaluate anatomy and esophageal motility and to assess for a hiatal hernia [5,8,32]. Fixed hiatal hernias or esophageal motility disorders may be associated with increased complications following LAGB, including band slippage and dysphasia [8,32].

Routine early postoperative UGI evaluation after LAGB is important to assess for extraluminal leak or obstruction. In addition, placement of the band, pouch size, and stoma size may be assessed [5,8,11,21,25,33]. Initially, a supine scout overhead radiograph is obtained to identify the location of the band, tubing, and port and to assess for contiguity of the connecting tubing (Fig. 2). To evaluate the Lap-Band system optimally, the patient is placed initially in the straight anteroposterior or slight right posterior oblique position to move the fundus to the left [8,33]. The patient is rotated at fluoroscopy so that the band is visualized in profile before administration of contrast material (Fig. 3A). This positioning allows optimal evaluation of the pouch and stoma (see Fig. 3) and is in contrast to the routine use of the left posterior oblique position for evaluating patients after RYGBP. In the left posterior oblique position after LAGB or if the band is visualized en face (Fig. 4A), the stoma is obscured quickly by contrast material within the fundus, precluding optimal postoperative evaluation of the pouch and stoma (Fig. 4).

In the early postoperative period, the author and colleagues routinely perform UGI examinations with water-soluble contrast material. If no leak is demonstrated, barium is administered. Contrast administration should reveal a small upper gastric pouch, a narrow stoma extending through the band, and opacification of the remainder of the stomach (see Fig. 3B; Fig. 5). There may be a mild delay in esophageal emptying, especially in the early postoperative course [8]. Although the band typically is left empty at surgery, postoperative edema may result in stomal narrowing [21].

Follow-up UGI examinations may be performed for vomiting, food intolerance, insufficient weight loss, excessive weight loss, epigastric pain, or at the time of planned adjustment procedures. For follow-up studies similar technique is used, but only barium is administered.

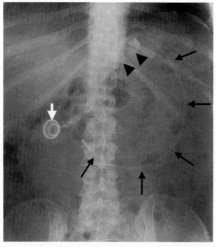

Fig. 2. Supine overhead radiograph shows the gastric band (*arrowheads*), the connecting tubing (*black arrows*), and the subcutaneous port (*white arrow*).

CT is not used routinely after LAGB and may not be technically feasible in the most severely obese patients; however, CT may be beneficial to evaluate for a source of infection and to assess for postoperative complications. LAGB also may be an incidental finding on CT performed for other indications. CT ideally is performed following both oral and intravenous contrast administration, and technical factors may need to be altered because of large patient size. CT images should reveal the radiopaque band around the proximal stomach and the attached connecting tubing extending through the anterior abdominal wall to the subcutaneous reservoir (Fig. 6).

## Fluoroscopic band adjustment

Fluoroscopic adjustment of the LAGB is performed most often by the radiologist in consultation with the surgeon based on the patient's ability to eat and the weight-loss curve [5,8,21,25,32,34]. The band system is left empty with the cuff deflated following surgery. Adjustments usually are performed around 6 weeks postoperatively, once edema has resolved [5,8,25]. UGI examinations should be performed both before and after the adjustment (Fig. 7) to avoid complications such as acute obstruction.

With the Lap-Band system, the stoma size is decreased by 0.5 mm following the addition of 0.4 $cm^3$ of saline; the maximal volume that can be injected into the band is 4 $cm^3$ [5,8]. The stoma optimally is calibrated to 3 to 5 mm in diameter, and the width of the stoma may be determined at UGI using the known diameter of the band [21,25,31].

The center of the subcutaneous port is localized at fluoroscopy. A radiopaque marker is placed on the skin (Fig. 7B). The skin is prepped with antiseptic solution, and local anesthesia is used. A 20- to 22-gauge noncoring, deflected-tip needle is used to access the port [8,21]. It is important to use a noncoring needle, because the wrong needle may damage the port and cause leakage from the system. In addition, puncture of the tubing rather than the port may cause leakage and device failure [8]. The noncoring needle with an attached saline-filled syringe is advanced until it hits the back wall of the reservoir (Fig. 7C). Saline can be easily withdrawn or injected to confirm appropriate position within the port. Saline then can be injected or withdrawn to decrease or increase the stomal size, respectively. The exact amount injected or withdrawn must be documented. Following the adjustment, contrast material must be administered orally to confirm adequate narrowing of the stoma without obstruction (Fig. 7D).

Approximately 3 to 3.5 $cm^3$ of saline must be added to the system to adjust the stoma to an

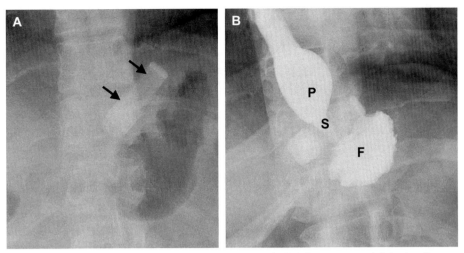

*Fig. 3.* Appropriate positioning for UGI following LAGB: optimal stomal assessment. (*A*) Supine fluoroscopic image obtained before contrast administration demonstrates appropriate patient positioning so that the band is imaged in profile (*arrows*) rather than as a ring shape. (*B*) Following administration of contrast material, the small gastric pouch (*P*) and narrow stoma through the band device (*S*) are well visualized. Contrast material passes through the narrow stoma (*S*) into the gastric fundus (*F*).

optimal 3- to 5-mm diameter [21]. Several adjustment procedures may be necessary. An average of three adjustments per patient may be required for adequate weight reduction [5,32]. Adjustments may be made using ultrasound guidance; however, UGI examinations still must be performed following band adjustment [34]. The use of fluoroscopy for stomal adjustments allows accurate adjustment of stomal size as well as reduction of complications from an excessively narrowed stoma that may

include obstruction, pouch enlargement, motility disorders, food intolerance, and band migration [32].

## Complications after laparoscopic adjustable gastric banding

LAGB is a safe procedure with minimal perioperative mortality [8,12,13,25]; however, some degree of morbidity may occur in up to 35% of patients [23]. Additional surgery may be necessary in 11%

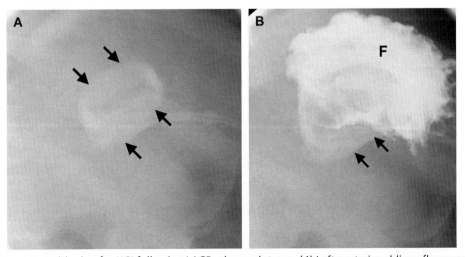

*Fig. 4.* Incorrect positioning for UGI following LAGB: obscured stoma. (*A*) Left posterior oblique fluoroscopic image obtained before contrast administration demonstrates incorrect patient positioning so that the band remains in a ringlike configuration (*arrows*). (*B*) Following administration of contrast material, the gastric fundus (*F*) is promptly opacified. In this position, contrast material in the fundus overlies the gastric band (*arrows*), and the stoma is not visualized.

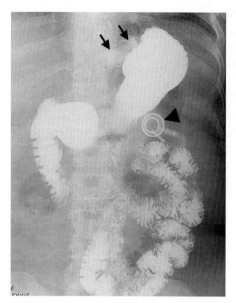

Fig. 5. Expected postoperative appearance following LAGB on UGI. A supine overhead radiograph from an UGI shows the radiopaque gastric band (*arrows*) and the subcutaneous reservoir (*arrowhead*). Contrast material is opacifying the remainder of the stomach, the duodenum, and the proximal small bowel.

of patients [12–15,23,31,35,36]. Most of the additional surgical procedures can be performed laparoscopically [12,37].

Early complications related to LAGB are rare. Gastroesophageal perforation occurs in less than 0.5% of patients [12,13,15,21,31]. Improper positioning of the band at surgery [21] and early

postoperative slippage of the band requiring repositioning each occur in less than 1% of patients [12–14,31]. Acute stomal obstruction may occur in 1.4% of patients and typically resolves spontaneously within a few days with conservative management [36]. Early dysphasia occurs in up to 14% of patients [25]. Regurgitation and pouch esophageal reflux are common until dietary habits change [21].

Late complications following LAGB are much more common than early postoperative complications. The most common long-term complications are pouch dilatation and slippage of the gastric band [21,23,25,31,38]. These complications require fluoroscopic contrast studies for diagnosis, and early diagnosis is crucial for success of the procedure [21,25]. Other significant late complications include intragastric band migration or erosion, acute obstruction, and device-related complications resulting in leakage of saline from the system or infection [6,12,13,15,21,25,31,33,36–39]. Gastric necrosis is a rare complication of LAGB (occurring in <0.3% of patients) that is most often due to slippage of the gastric band with subsequent strangulation [12,13,15].

### Pouch dilatation

A major long-term complication of LAGB is dilatation of the gastric pouch, occurring in up to 25% of patients [39]. However, pouch dilatation has decreased in incidence with recent modifications of the surgical procedure. Pouch dilatation can result in failed weight loss or stabilization of the weight loss curve and may require removal of the gastric band [24]. Pouch dilatation may occur with a normal

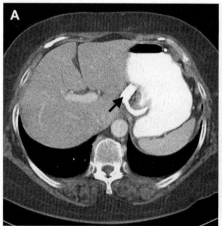
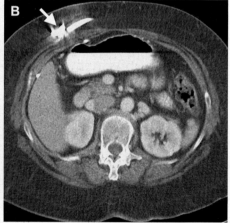

Fig. 6. Expected postoperative appearance following LAGB on CT. (*A*) Axial contrast-enhanced CT image shows the radiopaque gastric band (*arrow*) placed around the proximal stomach with attached connecting tubing. (*B*) Axial contrast-enhanced CT image more caudally shows the connecting tubing leading to the subcutaneous reservoir along the anterior rectus sheath (*arrow*).

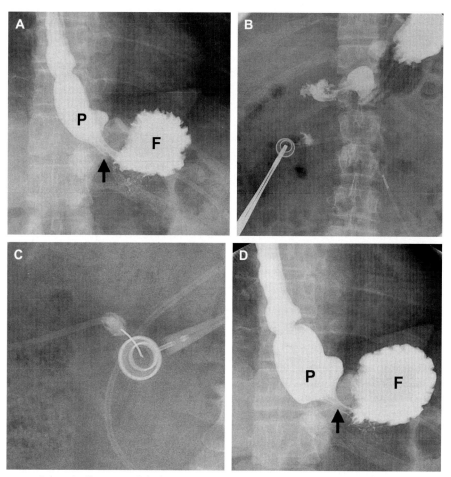

*Fig. 7.* Fluoroscopic band adjustment. (*A*) Fluoroscopic supine UGI image before adjustment shows the small gastric pouch (*P*), the stoma through the band (*arrow*) and the gastric fundus (*F*). The stoma measures 8 to 9 mm. (*B*) A fluoroscopic image shows localization of the reservoir and placement of a radiopaque marker over the reservoir. The site is marked subsequently on the skin, and the skin is prepped. (*C*) A fluoroscopic image shows advancement of a noncoring needle into the reservoir. (*D*) Fluoroscopic supine UGI image following adjustment of the band. Saline has been added to the inflatable cuff so that the stoma is narrower (*arrow*), measuring 4 to 5 mm. There is mild resultant dilatation of the gastric pouch (*P*). F, fundus.

or widened stoma, a stoma that is too narrow, or as a consequence of slippage of the gastric band.

*Concentric pouch dilatation with a normal or widened stoma*

Pouch dilatation may occur with a normal or widened stoma and usually results in chronic concentric dilatation of the gastric pouch [25]. This complication occurs most often as a result of dietary noncompliance and requires nutritional counseling [21,25]. In this scenario, chronic overfilling, rather than outflow obstruction, leads to pouch distention. At fluoroscopic examination, the stoma is within normal limits or actually widened, and the gastric pouch is dilated (Fig. 8). The large pouch allows further overeating and dilatation.

*Concentric pouch dilatation with a narrow stoma*

Pouch dilatation also may occur as a consequence of a stoma that is too narrow (Fig. 9). In this setting, concentric dilatation of the gastric pouch most often occurs acutely, as compared with the chronic dilatation that occurs with a normal-size stoma [21,25]. Patients may present with vomiting, dysphasia, esophageal dysmotility, pseudoachalasia, or obstruction [2,5].

Acute dilatation of the gastric pouch is most often caused by overinflation of the gastric band at the time of adjustment. Acute pouch dilatation also may be related to a focal weakness within the band with eccentric band herniation. Focal herniation of the band results in eccentric stomal

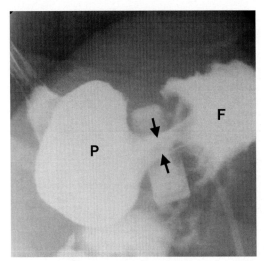

*Fig. 8.* Pouch dilatation with normal stoma. A fluoroscopic UGI image in a slight right posterior oblique position shows a normal-caliber stoma through the band (*arrows*). The pouch (*P*) is dilated concentrically. Contrast material is entering the gastric fundus (*F*).

narrowing, which may not be appreciated on UGI unless performed in different projections [21]. This problem can be diagnosed readily by filling the band with contrast material at fluoroscopy.

When pouch dilatation caused by stomal narrowing is identified, the band should be deflated immediately [5]. If diagnosed early, pouch dilatation may resolve with deflation of the band. If not diagnosed and treated promptly, pouch dilatation will recur despite deflation of the band in up to 50% of patients and may be irreversible [5]. Immediate

postadjustment UGI is important to prevent this complication.

### Eccentric pouch dilatation caused by band slippage

Eccentric pouch dilatation on UGI is most often a late complication following LAGB and is caused by slippage of the band. Dislocation of the band with herniation of a portion of the stomach above the band results in eccentric dilatation of the gastric pouch (Fig. 10). The complication of band slippage is discussed in more detail below.

### Band slippage

Band slippage occurs when the band is dislocated from its appropriate position. Herniation of the stomach above the band results in eccentric pouch enlargement [8,27]. Band slippage may result in failed weight loss and/or acute obstruction of the stoma [38]. Slippage of the gastric band is one of the most common complications following LAGB; the frequency depends on patient compliance, surgical technique, and postoperative care [25,29,38].

The incidence of band slippage varies most widely with the surgical technique used for placement of the band and has decreased substantially with surgical modifications over time [13,14,21,25, 28,33,36,39–43]. The incidence also may be decreased with patient training to encourage appropriate eating behaviors [39]. Overeating with overfilling of the gastric pouch, overinflation of the gastric band at the time of adjustments, and excessive vomiting are risk factors for band slippage [33,42,43]. Overall, band slippage occurs in up to

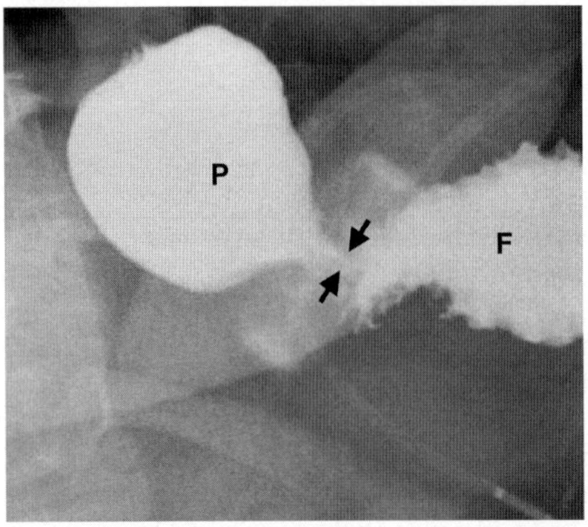

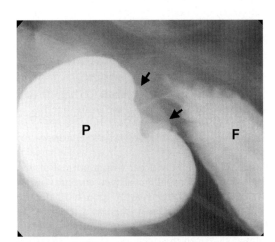

*Fig. 9.* Pouch dilatation with a narrow stoma. A fluoroscopic UGI image in a slight right posterior oblique position shows a narrow stoma (*arrows*), measuring only 2 to 3 mm, extending through the band. The pouch (*P*) is dilated concentrically. Contrast material is entering the gastric fundus (*F*).

*Fig. 10.* Pouch dilatation with band slippage. A fluoroscopic UGI image in a slight right posterior oblique position shows the band tilted and displaced (*arrows*) resulting in partial obstruction. There is eccentric dilatation of the gastric pouch (*P*) and a markedly narrowed stoma. F, fundus.

24% of patients [13,14,26,27,29,32,36,40]. Band slippage usually occurs as a late complication following LABG and has been diagnosed 3 to 58 months following surgery with a mean of 13.4 months [13,15,27,29,42].

Band slippage may be asymptomatic in up to 20% of patients, although patients also may present with acute food intolerance, epigastric pain, vomiting, progressive gastroesophageal reflux, esophageal motility disorders, or early satiety [15,27,42]. In a minority of patients, band slippage may produce sudden dysphasia and progressive severe upper abdominal pain [42]. Pouch dilatation and prolapse may cause complete dysphasia and acute gastric obstruction [8,42]. Slippage of the band also may result in ineffectiveness of the procedure with weight gain caused by pouch dilatation [38].

There are three different types of band slippage including anterior slippage, posterior slippage, and the most rare, concentric slippage with complete displacement of the band distally [27]. All three types of band slippage have similar consequences. Historically, posterior slippage occurred most commonly following LAGB, but rates have decreased dramatically with advances in surgical technique [2,13,28,36,40,43]. The incidence of posterior band slippage decreased in one study from 24% to 2% following surgical modifications [13]; however, despite surgical modifications, the incidence of posterior band slippage remains between 2% and 5% [13,42].

On the other hand, the incidence of anterior slippage remains relatively unchanged [2,29]. Anterior slippage is related to insufficient fixation of the band. At the time of surgery, nonabsorbable sutures are placed between the serosa proximal and distal to the band to maintain position and prevent anterior slippage along the high greater curvature. Failure to secure sutures properly or suture disruption allows distal slippage [43]. Predisposing factors for anterior band slippage include inadequate suture tension, suture disruption from overdistention/overfilling of the gastric pouch, overinflation of the gastric band, and/or excessive vomiting [29,43].

At UGI, a change in configuration of the band is noted when compared with the immediate postoperative study (**Fig. 11**). With anterior or posterior band slippage, the band is displaced into a more vertical or horizontal configuration, and there is resultant eccentric pouch dilatation (see **Figs. 10 and 11**) [13,21,25,43]. Gas within a distended gastric pouch may be noted on the scout overhead film (**Fig. 11C**), and the dilated gastric pouch may be located above or below the band [43]. Progressive eccentric pouch dilatation with herniation of the stomach above the band may occur if left untreated (**Fig. 11E**).

Intermittent slippage of the band also may result in chronic eccentric pouch dilatation [21]. In this setting, the band may slip back to a normal location following emptying of the gastric pouch or deflation of the system [21]. This situation may result in recurrent obstruction, because the band slips when the pouch is full.

Band slippage can lead to more severe complications including extreme eccentric pouch dilatation, obstruction at the site of the band, gastric volvulus, focal gastric ischemia, gastric infarction, perforation, and hemorrhage [21,43]. The most serious late complication of LAGB is necrosis of the gastric pouch [42]. Gastric necrosis is a rare, life-threatening complication of band slippage that may occur years after band placement [41,42]. The stomach distal to the band prolapses through the band, and infarction occurs because of the continuous pressure exerted by the band on the distended stomach with resultant decreased blood supply to the gastric wall. This occurrence often requires total gastrectomy [41]. Although the incidence of gastric necrosis is very low, once band slippage occurs, infarction may occur at any time [41].

Because slippage of the gastric band can be a severe, life-threatening complication of LAGB, early detection is essential [42]. Once band slippage is diagnosed, the band should be completely deflated immediately [8,42]. Deflation of the band may help temporarily, but surgical treatment with repositioning or replacing the band is necessary to prevent more dangerous complications [8,14,21,27,42,43].

### Intragastric migration of the band

Intragastric erosion, penetration, or migration of the band is an underreported major long-term complication following LAGB [6]. Migration of the band increases over time with long-term follow-up, probably related to the indwelling foreign body (ie, the gastric band) [13]. The reported prevalence of gastric band erosion ranges from 0 to 11%, with higher rates documented in studies with longer follow-up and in endoscopic studies [6,44]. More typical reported rates of band erosion following LAGB range from 0.2% to 2% [13,30,36,39,40,42,44,45].

With this complication, the gastric band gradually erodes or migrates into the gastric wall. After an initial tear, the band grows through the wall and may enter the gastric lumen (**Fig. 12**) [6,21]. This rare complication may be related to intraoperative damage to the outer gastric wall, the use of nonsteroidal anti-inflammatory medicines, excessive vomiting, increased pressure in the band caused by overinflation, or band infection [13,21]. Patients may present with nonspecific abdominal pain, gastrointestinal bleeding, intra-abdominal and/or port abscess, peritonitis,

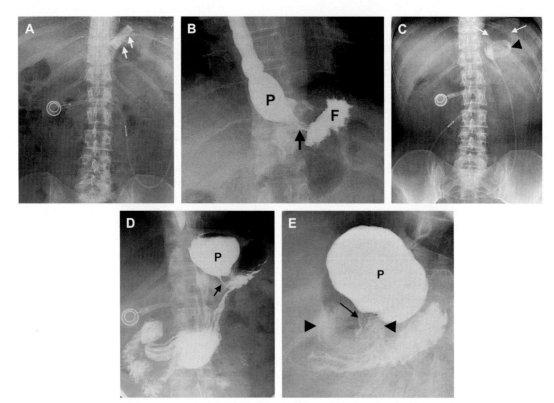

*Fig. 11.* Progressive band slippage. (*A*) A supine preliminary overhead radiograph in the early postoperative course shows appropriate positioning of the gastric band (*arrows*). (*B*) A supine fluoroscopic UGI image on the same day shows the small gastric pouch (*P*), the stoma through the band (*arrow*), and the gastric fundus (*F*). (*C*) A supine preliminary overhead radiograph obtained in the same patient 10 months later shows a change in configuration of the band with a more inferior and horizontal appearance (*arrowhead*). The gas-filled, dilated gastric pouch is located above the band (*arrows*). (*D*) A corresponding UGI image acquired in the upright position shows the dilated gastric pouch (*P*) above the displaced band with a markedly narrowed stoma (*arrow*). (*E*) A spot UGI image in the right posterior oblique position from a follow-up study performed 1 month later without interval intervention shows progressive eccentric dilatation of the gastric pouch (*P*) with inferior displacement of the band (*arrowheads*). The stoma is diminutive (*arrow*).

perforation, and, rarely, pneumoperitoneum [6,21,44–46]. Often, there is associated unexplained weight gain despite correct adjustment of the band [44].

Findings of band migration on UGI are pathognomonic. Contrast material is seen within the stoma and surrounding the part of the band that has migrated into the gastric lumen, so that the band appears as an intraluminal filling defect [6,21]. Knowledge of this complication is important, because there may be no extravasation of contrast material or other signs of perforation. CT may show extraluminal gas, peritoneal fluid, or abscess along the gastric wall or near the access port [6]. At endoscopy, there are three stages of band migration. In stage 1 a small part of the band is visible through a hole in the mucosa; in stage 2 there is partial migration with more than half of the band in the gastric lumen; in stage 3 there is complete migration of the band [44].

Band migration typically requires urgent surgical removal of the band and repair of the stomach, because erosion of the band can lead to fatal hemorrhage [6,21,44–46]. The band may be removed endoscopically if there has been partial or total migration [44].

## Problems with the port, connecting tubing, and band

Complications related to the reservoir, connecting tubing, or band itself have been reported in 1.4% to 26% of patients and in part depend on the length of follow-up [2,23,30,31,47]. Complications may include infection related to indwelling foreign bodies, leakage of saline from any part of the system with resultant band deflation, and migration or inversion of the port preventing band adjustments. These complications most often occur late and usually require surgical repair.

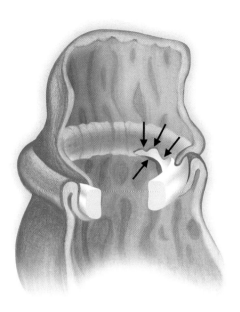

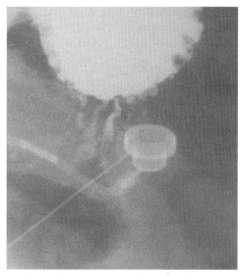

*Fig. 13.* Inverted reservoir. A fluoroscopic spot image from an attempted band adjustment shows inversion of the reservoir so that the needle cannot be advanced into the port.

*Fig. 12.* Migration of the gastric band into the lumen of the stomach. The diagram depicts the gastric band eroding into the gastric lumen. Arrows denote the tear in the gastric wall allowing migration of the band device into the gastric lumen.

Up to 11% of patients may require repeat surgery because of problems related to the reservoir [12,13,15,31,47]. The injectable port is sutured to the anterior rectus sheath. If sutures fail, the port may migrate, as has been reported in 0.4% of patients [8,12]. In addition, the port may become inverted or rotated in up to 3% of patients so that percutaneous puncture for band adjustments may not be possible (Fig. 13) [5,8,13,24,47]. Rotation or inversion of the port may be more common following major weight loss [13]. Rarely, an incisional hernia may develop at the port site [47].

Soft tissue infection involving the port and the band occurs in up to 6% and 3% of patients, respectively, and the incidence increases with length of follow-up [12,13,15,21,25,40,47]. Careful surgical technique may minimize infection. Also, the use of fluoroscopy and proper technique to perform adjustments minimizes failed punctures of the port and decreases damage and infection [47].

Leakage of saline from the system with spontaneous band deflation is a complication that may occur in up to 5% of patients and usually requires operative repair [4,5,13,21,33,47]. Band deflation results in a widened stoma, and patients experience a sudden change in dietary habits with associated weight gain [4,21,33,47]. Fluid loss from the system may be related to leakage from the port, from connecting tubing, or from the band itself [5,32]. Wear and tear around the port and tubing can lead to leakage and failure of the system. In most cases, fluid loss occurs at the reservoir. Leakage from the connecting tubing may occur as a consequence of inadvertent puncture of the tube at the time of adjustment [5,13]. In addition, the tubing may become disconnected.

If leakage from the system is suspected, an initial radiograph may be obtained to assess for acute angulation or disconnection of the connecting tube [5,33]. In addition, leakage from the system may be assessed by inserting a designated volume of saline into the port and measuring return upon deflation. A discrepancy in the returned volume implies leak [47]. Leakage from the port must be distinguished from leakage from the band or tube, because leakage from the port is easier to treat with local anesthesia in a simple surgical procedure [4]. Contrast injection of the port under fluoroscopy should distinguish leakage from the port, tubing, or adjustable balloon [4]. Water-soluble contrast material should be used to inject the port, because leakage from the system could be intraperitoneal in location [33].

Other reported problems related to the connecting tubing include intra-abdominal abscess, disconnection of tubing with migration into the small bowel, erosion of tubing into bowel as a consequence of wound infection with enterocutaneous fistula, and intracolonic penetration of the tubing [37,38,48].

### Esophageal dilatation and dysphasia

Initial experience with the Lap-Band system in the United States resulted in a high incidence of postoperative esophageal dilatation (Fig. 14) with vomiting, dysphagia, and/or reflux occurring in up to 72% of patients [22]. Progressive esophageal dilatation may lead to cessation of weight loss, because the patient no longer feels full [22]. More recent studies show a much lower incidence of esophageal dilatation, occurring in up to 2.4% of patients, likely related to advances in surgical technique [13,14].

Dysphagia is much more common in the early postoperative course and may occur in 14% of patients. Many of these patients improve over time without intervention or with dietary adjustments. Dysphagia also may develop as a late postoperative complication, requiring intervention in up to 6% of patients [25].

### Additional gastric complications

Acute gastric distension has been reported as an early complication following LAGB [49]. Patients who have diabetes and gastric dysmotility may be unable to decompress air trapped in the stomach, leading to severe acute distension. Nasogastric decompression and the use of promotility agents may relieve this condition [49]. A gastric bezoar may occur in up to 1.3% of patients at any time following LAGB [50]. Patients may present with persistent fullness, dysphagia, and vomiting. Endoscopic removal of the bezoar is often necessary. Diet modification with avoidance of high-residue cellulose foods and more complete mastication may prevent this complication.

### Summary

LAGB is a safe and effective means of weight loss in the morbidly obese patient population. Success of the procedure requires a team approach consisting of the surgeon, radiologist, and dietician. Patient compliance is also important for the success of the procedure. Many complications following LAGB are best diagnosed radiologically, and it is important for radiologists to be aware of the expected radiologic appearance, optimal technique for UGI examinations and stomal adjustments, and potential complications following LAGB. In addition, the radiologist often plays a crucial role in the management of weight loss and symptomatology in patients following LAGB by means of performing band adjustments.

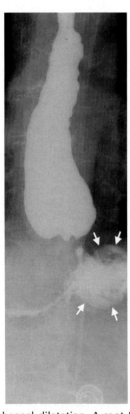

Fig. 14. Esophageal dilatation. A spot UGI image in the semi-upright, slight left posterior oblique position shows the gastric band obscured by contrast material in the stomach (*arrows*). There is esophageal dilation with a standing column of contrast material in the esophagus. Esophageal dysmotility also was noted at fluoroscopy.

### References

[1] Mognol P, Chosidow D, Marmuse JP. Laparoscopic gastric bypass versus laparoscopic adjustable gastric banding in the super-obese: a comparative study of 290 patients. Obes Surg 2005;15: 76–81.
[2] Watkins BM, Montgomery KF, Ahroni JH. Laparoscopic adjustable gastric banding: early experience in 400 consecutive patients in the USA. Obes Surg 2005;15:82–7.
[3] Mokdad AH, Bowman BA, Ford ES, et al. The continuing epidemics of obesity and diabetes in the United States. JAMA 2001;286:1195–200.
[4] Mittermair RP, Weiss HG, Nehoda H, et al. Band leakage after laparoscopic adjustable gastric banding. Obes Surg 2003;13:913–7.
[5] Hainaux B, Coppens E, Sattari A, et al. Laparoscopic adjustable silicone gastric banding: radiological appearances of a new surgical treatment for morbid obesity. Abdom Imaging 1999;24: 533–7.
[6] Hainaux B, Agneessens E, Rubesova E, et al. Intragastric band erosion after laparoscopic adjustable gastric banding for morbid obesity: imaging characteristics of an underreported complication. AJR Am J Roentgenol 2005;184:109–12.

[7] Chapman AE, Kiroff G, Game P, et al. Laparoscopic adjustable gastric banding in the treatment of obesity: a systematic literature review. Surgery 2004;135:326–51.

[8] Szucs RA, Turner MA, Kellum JM, et al. Adjustable laparoscopic gastric band for the treatment of morbid obesity: radiologic evaluation. AJR Am J Roentgenol 1998;170:993–6.

[9] National Institutes of Health Consensus Development Conference Statement. Gastrointestinal surgery for severe obesity: Am J Clin Nutr 1992; 55:615S–9S.

[10] Brolin RE. Update: NIH consensus conference. Gastrointestinal surgery for severe obesity. Nutrition 1996;12:403–4.

[11] Parikh MS, Laker S, Weiner M, et al. Objective comparison of complications resulting from laparoscopic bariatric procedures. J Am Coll Surg 2006;202:252–61.

[12] DeMaria EJ, Jamal MK. Laparoscopic adjustable gastric banding: evolving clinical experience. Surg Clin North Am 2005;85:773–87, vii.

[13] Chevallier JM, Zinzindohoue F, Douard R, et al. Complications after laparoscopic adjustable gastric banding for morbid obesity: experience with 1,000 patients over 7 years. Obes Surg 2004;14: 407–14.

[14] Weiner R, Blanco-Engert R, Weiner S, et al. Outcome after laparoscopic adjustable gastric banding—8 years experience. Obes Surg 2003;13:427–34.

[15] Zinzindohoue F, Chevallier JM, Douard R, et al. Laparoscopic gastric banding: a minimally invasive surgical treatment for morbid obesity: prospective study of 500 consecutive patients. Ann Surg 2003;237:1–9.

[16] Biertho L, Steffen R, Ricklin T, et al. Laparoscopic gastric bypass versus laparoscopic adjustable gastric banding: a comparative study of 1,200 cases. J Am Coll Surg 2003;197:536–44 [discussion: 544–5].

[17] Sarker S, Myers J, Serot J, et al. Three-year follow-up weight loss results for patients undergoing laparoscopic adjustable gastric banding at a major university medical center: does the weight loss persist? Am J Surg 2006;191:372–6.

[18] Kuzmak LI. A review of seven years' experience with silicone gastric banding. Obes Surg 1991; 1:403–8.

[19] Belachew M, Jacqet P, Lardinois F, et al. Vertical banded gastroplasty vs adjustable silicone gastric banding in the treatment of morbid obesity: a preliminary report. Obes Surg 1993;3:275–8.

[20] Cadiere GB, Bruyns J, Himpens J, et al. Laparoscopic gastroplasty for morbid obesity. Br J Surg 1994;81:1524.

[21] Wiesner W, Schob O, Hauser RS, et al. Adjustable laparoscopic gastric banding in patients with morbid obesity: radiographic management, results, and postoperative complications. Radiology 2000;216:389–94.

[22] DeMaria EJ, Sugerman HJ, Meador JG, et al. High failure rate after laparoscopic adjustable silicone gastric banding for treatment of morbid obesity. Ann Surg 2001;233:809–18.

[23] Suter M, Giusti V, Worreth M, et al. Laparoscopic gastric banding: a prospective, randomized study comparing the Lapband and the SAGB: early results. Ann Surg 2005;241:55–62.

[24] Mortele KJ, Pattijn P, Mollet P, et al. The Swedish laparoscopic adjustable gastric banding for morbid obesity: radiologic findings in 218 patients. AJR Am J Roentgenol 2001;177:77–84.

[25] Zacharoulis D, Roy-Chadhury SH, Dobbins B, et al. Laparoscopic adjustable gastric banding: surgical and radiological approach. Obes Surg 2002;12:280–4.

[26] Srikanth MS, Oh KH, Keskey T, et al. Critical extreme anterior slippage (paragastric Richter's hernia) of the stomach after laparoscopic adjustable gastric banding: early recognition and prevention of gastric strangulation. Obes Surg 2005;15: 207–15 [discussion: 215].

[27] Wolnerhanssen B, Kern B, Peters T, et al. Reduction in slippage with 11-cm Lap-Band and change of gastric banding technique. Obes Surg 2005; 15:1050–4.

[28] Rubin M, Benchetrit S, Lustigman H, et al. Laparoscopic gastric banding with Lap-Band for morbid obesity: two-step technique may improve outcome. Obes Surg 2001;11:315–7.

[29] Weiner R, Bockhorn H, Rosenthal R, et al. A prospective randomized trial of different laparoscopic gastric banding techniques for morbid obesity. Surg Endosc 2001;15:63–8.

[30] Angrisani L, Alkilani M, Basso N, et al. Laparoscopic Italian experience with the Lap-Band. Obes Surg 2001;11:307–10.

[31] Favretti F, Cadiere GB, Segato G, et al. Laparoscopic banding: selection and technique in 830 patients. Obes Surg 2002;12:385–90.

[32] Frigg A, Peterli R, Zynamon A, et al. Radiologic and endoscopic evaluation for laparoscopic adjustable gastric banding: preoperative and follow-up. Obes Surg 2001;11:594–9.

[33] Pomerri F, De Marchi F, Barbiero G, et al. Radiology for laparoscopic adjustable gastric banding: a simplified follow-up examination method. Obes Surg 2003;13:901–8.

[34] Pretolesi F, Camerini G, Bonifacino E, et al. Radiology of adjustable silicone gastric banding for morbid obesity. Br J Radiol 1998;71:717–22.

[35] Abu-Abeid S, Szold A. Results and complications of laparoscopic adjustable gastric banding: an early and intermediate experience. Obes Surg 1999;9:188–90.

[36] Ponce J, Paynter S, Fromm R. Laparoscopic adjustable gastric banding: 1,014 consecutive cases. J Am Coll Surg 2005;201:529–35.

[37] Zengin K, Sen B, Ozben V, et al. Detachment of the connecting tube from the port and migration into jejunal wall. Obes Surg 2006;16:206–7.

[38] Hartmann J, Scharfenberg M, Paul M, et al. Intracolonic penetration of the laparoscopic adjustable gastric banding tube. Obes Surg 2006;16:203–5.

[39] Zappa MA, Micheletto G, Lattuada E, et al. Prevention of pouch dilatation after laparoscopic adjustable gastric banding. Obes Surg 2006;16:132–6.

[40] Capizzi FD, Boschi S, Brulatti M, et al. Laparoscopic adjustable esophagogastric banding: preliminary results. Obes Surg 2002;12:391–4.

[41] Iannelli A, Facchiano E, Sejor E, et al. Gastric necrosis: a rare complication of gastric banding. Obes Surg 2005;15:1211–4.

[42] Kriwanek S, Schermann M, Ali Abdullah S, et al. Band slippage—a potentially life-threatening complication after laparoscopic adjustable gastric banding. Obes Surg 2005;15:133–6.

[43] Wiesner W, Weber M, Hauser RS, et al. Anterior versus posterior slippage: two different types of eccentric pouch dilatation in patients with adjustable laparoscopic gastric banding. Dig Surg 2001;18:182–6 [discussion: 187].

[44] Nocca D, Frering V, Gallix B, et al. Migration of adjustable gastric banding from a cohort study of 4236 patients. Surg Endosc 2005;19:947–50.

[45] Abu-Abeid S, Bar Zohar D, Sagie B, et al. Treatment of intra-gastric band migration following laparoscopic banding: safety and feasibility of simultaneous laparoscopic band removal and replacement. Obes Surg 2005;15:849–52.

[46] Wylezol M, Sitkiewicz T, Gluck M, et al. Intra-abdominal abscess in the course of intragastric migration of an adjustable gastric band: a potentially life-threatening complication. Obes Surg 2006;16:102–4.

[47] Keidar A, Carmon E, Szold A, et al. Port complications following laparoscopic adjustable gastric banding for morbid obesity. Obes Surg 2005;15:361–5.

[48] Elakkary E, El Essawy D, Gazayerli MM. Enterocutaneous fistula: a rare complication of laparoscopic adjustable gastric banding. Obes Surg 2005;15:897–900.

[49] Shayani V, Sarker S. Diagnosis and management of acute gastric distention following laparoscopic adjustable gastric banding. Obes Surg 2004;14:702–4.

[50] Veronelli A, Ranieri R, Laneri M, et al. Gastric bezoars after adjustable gastric banding. Obes Surg 2004;14:796–7.

ELSEVIER
SAUNDERS

RADIOLOGIC
CLINICS
OF NORTH AMERICA

Radiol Clin N Am 45 (2007) 275–288

# Multidetector CT Angiography in the Diagnosis of Mesenteric Ischemia

Karen M. Horton, MD*, Elliot K. Fishman, MD

- CT protocol
  *Oral contrast medium*
  *Intravenous contrast medium*
  *Scan parameters*
  *3D imaging and image review*
- Vascular anatomy

- Acute mesenteric ischemia
  *CT findings*
- Chronic mesenteric ischemia
  *Diagnosis*
- Summary
- References

Multidetector CT (MDCT) is an ideal tool for the diagnosis of acute and chronic mesenteric ischemia. It is relatively noninvasive, requiring only a peripheral intravenous catheter for delivery of iodinated contrast material. It can be performed quickly and in a wide range of patients, including those who are critically ill. Because of rapid technological advances in both scanners and computer workstations, MDCT in many cases has replaced conventional catheter angiography for evaluation of the mesenteric vasculature and bowel.

CT angiography (CTA) yields volume data sets that can be reformatted and viewed in any projection, visualizing even tiny distal vascular segments and depicting stenosis and also its cause, including atherosclerotic plaque, thrombus, tumor, and anatomic abnormalities. Moreover, MDCT enables detailed evaluation of each bowel segment for evidence of ischemia or infarction.

Advanced CT scanners and expertise in three-dimensional (3D) imaging are becoming increasingly widespread, opening the door to new opportunities and challenges in the evaluation of patients suspected of having mesenteric ischemia. This article reviews contrast administration and image acquisition protocols, the anatomy of the mesenteric vasculature, the etiology of acute and chronic mesenteric ischemia, and CT findings diagnostic for these conditions.

## CT protocol

### Oral contrast medium

MDCT imaging of the mesenteric vessels and small intestine requires careful attention to the selection of oral contrast material. Abdominal CT traditionally has involved the use of positive oral contrast agents, which appear white on the CT scan. Positive agents include barium suspensions such as barium sulfate and, more recently, iodinated solutions such as diatrizoate sodium and iohexol.

Although positive oral contrast agents are acceptable for use in routine abdominal CT, their utility is limited for the detailed examination of the small bowel and mesenteric vessels. Intravenous contrast material causes the small bowel wall and mesenteric arteries to enhance brightly and appear white. Simultaneous use of an oral contrast agent that produces white intraluminal contents obscures the distinction between the bowel wall and the lumen and complicates 3D visualization of the mesenteric vessels [1].

Johns Hopkins Medical Institutions, 601 N. Caroline Street/JHOC 3253, Baltimore, MD 21287, USA
* Corresponding author.
*E-mail address:* kmhorton@jhmi.edu (K.M. Horton).

0033-8389/07/$ – see front matter © 2007 Elsevier Inc. All rights reserved.       doi:10.1016/j.rcl.2007.03.010
radiologic.theclinics.com

Negative contrast agents are one alternative [2,3]. Fat-based negative contrast agents have the dual advantages of emptying slowly from the stomach and producing low-attenuation intraluminal contents. They have practical limitations, however. Most patients are unwilling to drink large quantities of corn oil, for example. Whole milk, with a fat content of 4%, is another option. Thompson and coworkers [4] reported that whole milk produced excellent gastrointestinal distention, mural visualization, and bowel loop discrimination. Although milk is more palatable than corn oil, many patients cannot tolerate large quantities. Carbon dioxide is another potentially useful negative contrast agent, but it cannot be delivered noninvasively to the bowel [5].

Most radiologists, therefore, use a neutral contrast agent when examining the small intestine and mesenteric vessels. Neutral oral contrast agents include water, methylcellulose solutions, polyethylene glycol solutions, and very dilute barium solutions. By producing low-density intraluminal contents, neutral contrast agents improve visualization of the brightly enhancing bowel wall and obviate editing of the bowel for examination of the mesenteric vessels.

Megibow and coworkers [6] recently compared the neutral oral contrast agents VoLumen (E-Z-EM, Westbury, New York) and methylcellulose in 60 patients undergoing CT of the pancreas. Half of the patients consumed 1200 mL of VoLumen over 30 minutes, and the other half consumed a 3:1 mixture of water and methylcellulose over the same time period. The dilute barium agent, which had an attenuation of only 20 to 40 Hounsfield units, resulted in superior distention of the bowel and demonstration of mural features. Future studies will provide additional comparative data to guide the selection of neutral oral contrast agents for CT applications.

At Johns Hopkins Medical Institutions, water is used as the neutral oral contrast agent when imaging the small intestine and mesenteric vessels. Among its advantages are its low cost and ready acceptance by patients. One disadvantage of water is its rapid emptying from the stomach. Therefore, patients typically consume 750 to 1000 mL of water 30 minutes before the CT examination and an additional 250 mL immediately before scanning to ensure that the stomach and duodenum are distended.

Because water is absorbed readily by the small intestine, distention of the terminal ileum may be suboptimal. Intravenous glucagon is one option for improving bowel distention; however, rapid intravenous injection of a bolus of contrast material results in excellent visualization of the enhancing bowel wall, even in the case of incomplete bowel distention.

### Intravenous contrast medium

Rapid injection of intravenous contrast material, in combination with a dual-phase image acquisition protocol, ensures excellent visualization of both the mesenteric arteries and the mesenteric veins. At Johns Hopkins, 120 mL of nonionic contrast material is injected at 3 to 5 mL/s through a peripheral intravenous catheter line, typically an 18- or 20-gauge angiocatheter in the antecubital fossa. The arterial-phase acquisition takes place 30 seconds after the injection of contrast material, and the venous-phase acquisition 60 seconds after the contrast injection. For routine studies the authors use iohexol. In patients who have renal insufficiency, they use isosmolar contrast, iodixanol.

### Scan parameters

A CT scan of the small intestine and mesenteric vessels spans from the diaphragm through the symphysis pubis. Mesenteric arteries are very small, with distal branches measuring 1 mm or less in diameter. It is critical, therefore, that the CT scan be performed using the thinnest possible collimation, typically 0.75 mm on a 16-slice scanner and 0.6 mm on a 64-slice scanner. The use of 0.75-mm overlapping slices and a reconstruction interval of 0.5 mm produces a volume data set that is ideal for 3D imaging.

Data also may be reconstructed in 3- to 5-mm slices for review of other abdominal organs on a picture archiving and communications system or on film, without the grainy appearance associated with very-thin-slice axial reconstructions. Therefore, each data set is reconstructed twice. The thin slices are used for 3D imaging, and the thick slices are used for review of the other organs. A 120 kilovolts (kV) and 270 effective milliamperes (mAs) are usually adequate.

### 3D imaging and image review

A comprehensive CT examination in patients suspected of having mesenteric ischemia requires review of both the vasculature and the bowel. Initial evaluation of the CT data set generally begins with scrolling through the thin axial images to evaluate proximal arterial patency. A sagittal projection is most useful when evaluating the origin and proximal portions of the mesenteric arteries and for identifying anatomic variants (Fig. 1A). Evaluation with volume rendering in a coronal or coronal oblique projection enables detailed evaluation of branch vessels, even tiny distal branches (Fig. 1B). The smallest branches are often best appreciated with a maximum intensity projection (MIP) (Fig. 1C).

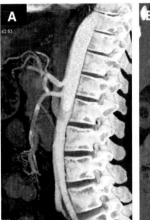
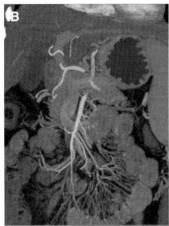
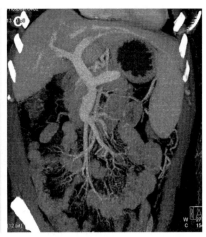

*Fig. 1.* (*A*) Sagittal volume-rendered 3D CTA demonstrates the normal anatomy of the celiac axis and SMA. The origin and proximal segment of these vessels is best appreciated in the sagittal projection. (*B*) Coronal volume-rendered 3D CTA demonstrates the normal branching pattern of the SMA. Distal branches of the SMA are visualized best in the coronal projection using either volume rendering or MIP. (*C*) Coronal MIP image demonstrates the normal anatomy of the mesenteric veins.

The venous data set is reviewed using a similar approach. Examination of the mesenteric veins is accomplished best using a coronal or coronal oblique projection using a combination of MIP and volume rendering (see Fig. 1). 3D review of both the arterial and venous data sets typically takes approximately 5 minutes.

Examination of the small bowel loops in the axial plane usually is difficult and ineffective. Instead, a coronal projection is preferred for a comprehensive visualization of the entire small intestine. This visualization can be done with a combination of multiplanar reformation (MPR) or volume rendering using clip planes (Fig. 2). Clip planes enable

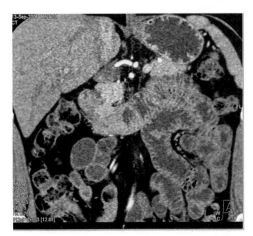

*Fig. 2.* Thin-slab coronal volume-rendered image demonstrates the normal appearance of the small bowel when water is used as oral contrast. Individual small bowel folds are often visible.

examination of each of the many folds in the duodenum and jejunum, observation of the transition to the ileum, where there are fewer folds, and close examination of the terminal ileum as it comes into the ileocecal valve.

## Vascular anatomy

Evaluation of the mesenteric vessels requires a detailed understanding of vascular anatomy. Three main arteries supply blood to the gut. The first is the celiac axis, which supplies the foregut, from the distal esophagus through the second portion of the duodenum. The proximal branch vessels off the celiac axis are the common hepatic, splenic, and left gastric arteries. The gastroduodenal artery is the first branch off the common hepatic artery.

The second major artery supplying the gut is the superior mesenteric artery (SMA). The SMA supplies the midgut, consisting of the third and fourth portions of the duodenum, the jejunum, ileum, right colon, and the transverse colon to approximately the splenic flexure.

The third major artery, the inferior mesenteric artery (IMA), supplies the colon from approximately the splenic flexure to the rectum. It has several branches: the left colic, marginal, sigmoid, and superior hemorrhoidal arteries.

There are also several common collateral pathways that maintain blood flow to the gut in the case of arterial stenosis or occlusion. The gastroduodenal artery, for example, is an important collateral pathway between the celiac axis and the SMA. In a patient who has stenosis at the origin of the celiac axis, CT typically demonstrates a dilated gastroduodenal artery, because blood flows through the SMA and the gastroduodenal artery to the common hepatic artery. Blood can flow in either direction, however, depending on the site of the occlusion.

The most significant collateral pathways between the SMA and IMA are the marginal artery of Drummond and the arc of Riolan (or paracolic arcade). These vessels typically appear dilated in a patient who has stenosis of the SMA, because blood flows from the IMA to the SMA, or vice versa. In addition, there are important collateral pathways between the IMA and the systemic circulation. For example, in a patient who has stenosis of the IMA, blood flow often is redirected through its hemorrhoidal branches to the sacral and internal iliac arteries.

Normal anatomic variants of the mesenteric arteries include a celiac axis and SMA arising from a single trunk of the abdominal aorta and a right hepatic artery arising from the SMA rather than the celiac axis. In approximately 15% of patients, the median arcuate ligament—the fibrous arch that unites the crura on either side of the diaphragm—crosses the aorta lower than usual, causing a small kink in the celiac axis [7,8]. In most cases, this kink represents a normal anatomic variant; however, in a small percentage of patients, low insertion of the median arcuate ligament causes significant stenosis of the proximal portion of the celiac axis, a condition known as "median arcuate ligament syndrome." Typically the stenosis is worse on expiration [9]. Given that CT is performed on inspiration, observation of any stenosis may be important, especially in symptomatic patients (Fig. 3) [10]. The diagnosis remains controversial, however [11].

Evaluation of the mesenteric vasculature involves the veins as well as the mesenteric arteries. Blood from the intestine flows through the superior mesenteric vein (SMV) and inferior mesenteric vein,

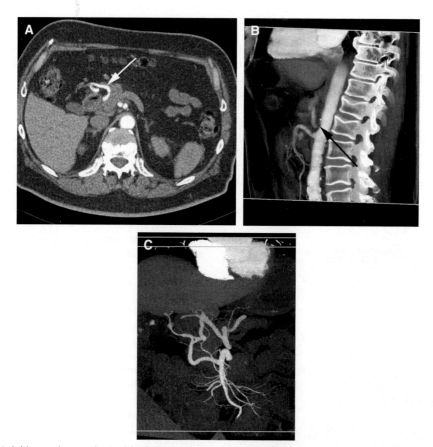

Fig. 3. (A) Axial image in a patient with abdominal pain demonstrates a prominent vessel (*arrow*) near the pancreatic head. This finding often is an indication that there may be a stenosis in the proximal celiac artery or SMA (as shown in Fig. 3B). (B) Sagittal volume-rendered 3D CTA demonstrates the stenosis of the proximal celiac axis (*arrow*). Notice the classic hooked appearance. This figure is an example of surgically proven median arcuate ligament syndrome. (C) Coronal MIP image shows a common collateral pathway between the SMA and celiac axis. The gastroduodenal artery supplies blood to the celiac axis distal to the stenosis.

which in most cases joins the splenic vein. Together the SMV and splenic vein supply blood to the portal vein and, ultimately, the liver.

Normal anatomic variants include a confluence of the inferior mesenteric vein with the SMV rather than the splenic vein. In addition, the angle at which the SMV and splenic vein join the portal vein varies, generally without clinical significance.

## Acute mesenteric ischemia

In a resting state, approximately 20% of cardiac output is delivered to the small intestine, whereas after a meal blood flow to the small intestine increases to approximately 35% of cardiac output. Mesenteric ischemia is a complex disorder caused by any of several conditions that reduce blood flow to the intestines. It can be acute or chronic and increases in incidence with age.

Acute mesenteric ischemia accounts for nearly 1 in 100 hospital admissions [12,13]. Despite advances in diagnosis and treatment, mortality remains as high as 70% [14]. Mesenteric ischemia can be caused by arterial or venous compromise or by a low-flow state. In 60% to 70% of cases, the cause of acute mesenteric ischemia is occlusion of the SMA by either an embolism or thrombus. In 20% to 30% of cases, the cause is nonocclusive—a low-flow state caused by hypotension or certain medications. In 5% to 10% of cases, acute mesenteric ischemia is caused by thrombosis of the mesenteric vein [12].

Although early recognition and treatment of acute mesenteric ischemia are critical, the diagnosis of this condition is difficult. The clinical presentation of acute mesenteric ischemia is nonspecific. Patients complain of abdominal pain, but its intensity often is out of proportion to an unremarkable physical examination. Blood levels of lactic acid may be elevated, as may be the white blood cell count and sedimentation rate. There are no laboratory tests that definitively diagnose acute mesenteric ischemia, however.

Conventional catheter angiography is considered the criterion for the diagnosis of mesenteric ischemia, but it is invasive and is not always ordered in a timely fashion. Multidetector CTA is an ideal alternative: it is minimally invasive, requiring only a peripheral intravenous catheter for injection of contrast medium. Moreover, it can be completed in a few minutes, improving the efficiency of diagnosis and minimizing the time critically ill patients spend in the scanner.

Most important, multidetector CTA is highly accurate. Kirkpatrick and coworkers [15] found that CTA had a sensitivity of 96% and a specificity of 94% for the diagnosis of acute mesenteric ischemia. As a result, the clinician can confidently send the patient for surgery or interventional therapy if the CT scan is positive for ischemia or can rule out ischemia and pursue another diagnosis if the bowel and blood vessels appear normal on CT.

## CT findings

### Bowel thickening

Ischemia usually causes circumferential thickening of the bowel wall [16]. Whereas the normal small bowel wall is less than 3 mm thick when adequately distended, an ischemic bowel wall is typically 8 to 9 mm thick and in some cases becomes as thick as 1.5 cm. Bowel wall thickening is more pronounced in cases of venous thrombosis than in cases of arterial thrombosis [17]. Therefore, in the setting of suspected ischemia, a bowel wall measuring 1.5 cm thick probably signals obstruction of venous blood flow (Fig. 4). Rapid contrast delivery results in dramatic early small bowel enhancement. This normal blush of enhancement should not be mistaken for small bowel thickening [1]. Arterial obstruction, particularly transmural infarction, usually manifests as a paper-thin bowel wall, the result of the destruction of muscle and nerve tissue (Fig. 5) [18]. Therefore, although thickening of the small bowel wall is a common finding, the presence and degree of thickening does not necessarily correlate with the severity of the ischemic damage [19].

### Bowel dilatation

Bowel dilatation is another common finding, but it is not specific for mesenteric ischemia [16]. Severe dilatation is most common with irreversible transmural ischemia or infarction, which disrupts normal peristalsis (see Fig. 5) [18,20].

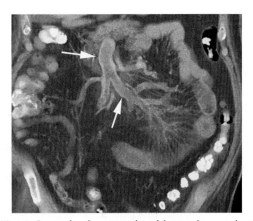

**Fig. 4.** Coronal volume-rendered image in a patient presenting with acute abdominal pain demonstrates extensive thrombosis (*arrows*) of the mesenteric veins. The proximal jejunum is thickened, and there also is mesenteric stranding.

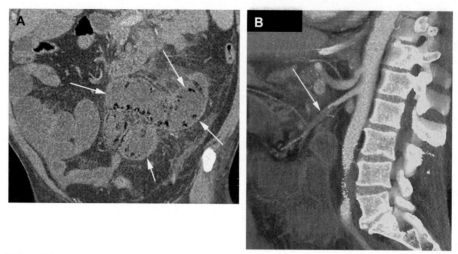

*Fig. 5.* (*A*) Thin-slab coronal volume-rendered image in a patient with acute abdominal pain and elevated lactic acid shows dilated small bowel loops with pneumatosis (*arrows*). The small bowel wall is not thickened. (*B*) Sagittal volume-rendered 3D CTA demonstrates a large thrombus (*arrow*) in the SMA. This is a common location for emboli to lodge.

### Bowel wall attenuation

In addition to bowel wall thickening and dilatation, it is important to assess bowel wall attenuation [1,21]. A low-density bowel wall is indicative of edema. In addition, several layers of submucosal edema and inflammation may create a characteristic halo effect. A high-density bowel wall can be the result of hemorrhage, either submucosal or transmural [21].

Pneumatosis is associated with air in the bowel wall (Fig. 6A). This sign of mucosal disruption usually is indicative of infarction. Pneumatosis is seen in 6% to 30% of patients who have acute mesenteric ischemia [18,22,23] and results from the extension of air from the bowel lumen into the wall. Further extension of air into the mesenteric

veins and, ultimately, the portal vein is known as portomesenteric gas and is observed in 3% to 14% of cases (Fig. 6B) [24]. Pneumatosis does not always indicate transmural infarction; however, patients who have pneumatosis and associated portomesenteric venous gas are more likely to have transmural infarction than those who have pneumatosis alone [24].

In some cases, it is possible to observe abnormalities in the pattern of bowel wall enhancement [22]. Delayed enhancement on early-phase imaging and persistent enhancement on late-phase imaging may aid in the identification of ischemic bowel segments. A complete lack of enhancement is highly specific for bowel infarction. It is an uncommon finding, however, because the redundancy of

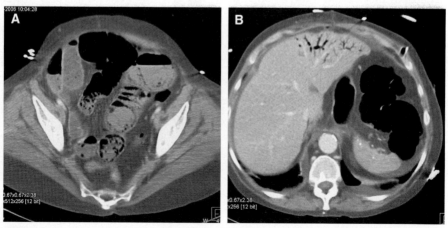

*Fig. 6.* (*A*) Axial image through the pelvis in a patient who has mesenteric ischemia shows small bowel pneumatosis. (*B*) Axial image through the liver in the same patient shows portal venous gas in the liver.

mesenteric vessels ensures that contrast is delivered even to very ischemic regions. Hyperemia also can occur after the administration of intravenous contrast medium and has been reported to have a sensitivity of 33% and a specificity of 71% for acute mesenteric ischemia [22]. The presence of hyperemia may be a good prognostic sign, because it probably indicates viable bowel.

### Mesenteric edema

CT also may demonstrate stranding and ascites. These findings are nonspecific, however. Their presence depends on the cause, severity, and duration of mesenteric ischemia [19].

### Vascular findings

**Arterial thrombus/emboli.** Vascular CT findings in acute mesenteric ischemia include embolism or thrombus in the mesenteric arteries or veins and atherosclerotic plaque, which can be a focus on which thrombus forms.

Emboli to the SMA usually originate in the heart or aorta and lodge 3 to 10 cm from the origin of the artery (see Fig. 5). In most cases, blood flow is preserved to the proximal branches of the SMA and to the jejunal and middle colic arteries [25]. Smaller emboli lodge more distally and affect only small segments of bowel. Therefore, it is important to carefully examine each bowel loop for evidence of ischemia or infarction.

Thrombosis of the SMA usually occurs in the setting of atherosclerotic disease. Indeed, 80% of patients who have SMA thrombosis have a history of chronic mesenteric ischemia marked by repeated episodes of abdominal pain [26]. The patient then presents with symptoms of acute mesenteric ischemia, probably resulting from the rupture of an unstable atherosclerotic plaque. Unlike emboli, thrombi typically develop at the origin of the SMA.

Traditionally, therapy for acute mesenteric ischemia consisted of exploratory laparotomy with resection of the nonviable bowel and re-establishment of blood flow to the intestines. Recent advances in interventional radiology offer effective, less invasive therapeutic alternatives. Intra-arterial thrombolysis, angioplasty, and stent placement are all available and effective [27].

**Vasculitis.** Vasculitis is another cause of acute mesenteric ischemia and can be divided into three categories: large-, medium-, and small-vessel vasculitis. Involvement of the mesenteric arteries can result in pain, acute or chronic mesenteric ischemia, hemorrhage, and/or stricture. The most common large-vessel vasculitis affecting the mesenteric vessels is Takayasu vasculitis [28], which targets the aorta and its major branches. The most common medium-vessel vasculitis is polyarteritis nodosum [29], a necrotizing form of the disease that weakens the vessel wall and can cause the formation of aneurysms. Some 80% to 90% of cases involve the kidneys and renal arteries; approximately 50% of cases involve the small intestine and mesenteric vessels. The most common vasculidities to involve the small intestine are Henoch-Schönlein purpura, systemic lupus erythematosus, and Behçet's disease [30–34].

On CT, small bowel vasculitis can appear as bowel thickening, edema, ulceration, and pruning of the mesenteric arteries (Fig. 7).

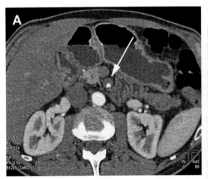 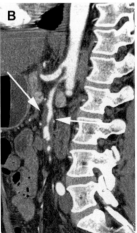 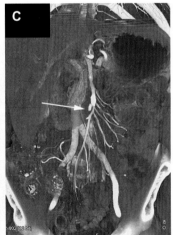

*Fig. 7.* (*A*) Axial CT in a 45-year-old patient with recurrent abdominal pain shows marked mural thickening of the SMA (*arrow*). (*B*) Sagittal MPR shows the extensive thickening along the proximal SMA (*arrows*). (*C*) Coronal volume-rendered 3D CTA shows the irregularity in the SMA and a small pseudoaneurysm (*arrow*). Based on the CT diagnosis of vasculitis, the patient was treated successfully with steroids.

**Dissection.** Dissection of the SMA is another cause of acute mesenteric ischemia, in most cases resulting from an aortic dissection that extends into the mesenteric vessel (Fig. 8). Isolated SMA dissection is very rare [35] and is thought to result from cystic medial necrosis and fibrous dysplasia. The clinical symptoms of SMA dissection are related to intestinal ischemia and hemorrhage.

**Aneurysm.** Splanchnic artery aneurysms, both true aneurysms and pseudoaneurysms, represent another cause of mesenteric ischemia, albeit a rare one. The overall incidence of splanchnic artery aneurysms is low (0.01%–0.25% at autopsy). The splenic artery is the most common site (60%), followed by the hepatic artery (20%), SMA (6%), celiac artery (4%), pancreaticoduodenal artery (2%), and gastroduodenal artery (1.5%) [36]. Splanchnic artery aneurysms may cause abdominal pain, bleeding, and rupture. In most cases, however, the aneurysm is detected incidentally in asymptomatic patients during cross-sectional imaging (Fig. 9) [37].

**Venous thrombosis.** Acute mesenteric ischemia also can result from thrombosis of the SMV (see Fig. 4; Fig. 10). Nearly 50% of patients who have SMV thrombosis have a personal or family history consistent with a hypercoagulable state, including pulmonary embolism or deep venous thrombosis [38]. Tumor encasement and inflammatory conditions such as diverticulitis can also cause mesenteric vein thrombosis.

The symptoms of mesenteric vein thrombosis are less acute than those associated with arterial occlusion, and patients often experience symptoms for as long as a month before seeking medical attention [39]. Mortality is as high as 40% [40]. CT findings include thrombus in the SMV and diffuse thickening of the small bowel and right colon. The bowel also may have a halo appearance as a result of submucosal edema. Venous thrombosis can be treated with systemic anticoagulation or percutaneous transhepatic delivery of thrombolytic agents [27].

**Low-flow states.** A low-flow state or hypotension can cause acute mesenteric ischemia, often in association with shock [41]. Other conditions that may precipitate a low-flow state are heart failure, hypovolemia, dehydration, and chronic renal failure, particularly after dialysis [42]. Certain drugs, such as digitalis, norepinephrine, cocaine, and ergot derivatives, also are known to cause low-flow states [27]. Patients present with abdominal distention and in some cases gastrointestinal bleeding, but they seldom complain of severe abdominal pain. CT typically shows diffuse thickening of the bowel. Blood vessels are small and pruned down, a result of the body's attempt to maintain blood flow to the gut (Fig. 11). Nonocclusive mesenteric ischemia often can be treated with selective arterial administration of vasodilating agents (ie, papaverine) [27].

## Chronic mesenteric ischemia

Chronic mesenteric ischemia, also known as abdominal angina, is caused by chronic arterial insufficiency of the intestines resulting from atherosclerotic disease of the mesenteric vessels. It is an uncommon but important cause of abdominal pain in elderly patients. Chronic mesenteric ischemia accounts for approximately 5% of all ischemic intestinal illnesses but results in significant morbidity and mortality [43].

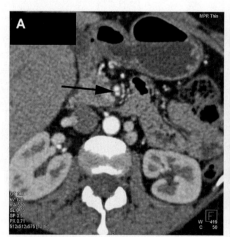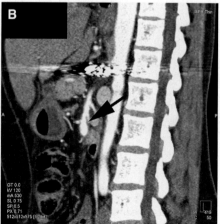

*Fig. 8.* (*A*) Axial image demonstrates an isolated dissection of the SMA (*arrow*). (*B*) Sagittal MPR also demonstrates the focal dissection flap (*arrow*). Notice that there is no aortic dissection.

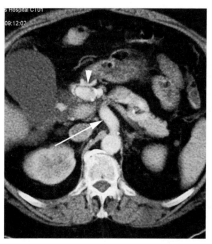

Fig. 9. Axial image shows a dilated celiac axis (*arrow*) as well as a focal aneurysm of the common hepatic artery (*arrowhead*).

The mean age of patients who have chronic mesenteric ischemia is 60 years [44]. Women are three times as likely as men to develop the disease. The incidence of chronic mesenteric ischemia is also higher in smokers and those who have other risk factors for atherosclerotic disease, such as diabetes. One third of patients have hypertension [45].

The detection of calcified atherosclerotic plaque on CT is not in itself diagnostic for chronic mesenteric ischemia (Fig. 12). In fact, atherosclerotic disease of the mesenteric vessels is a common incidental finding in asymptomatic elderly patients [46,47]. It is important, however, to document the presence of atherosclerotic plaque in the report to clinicians and to quantify the degree of stenosis, if possible.

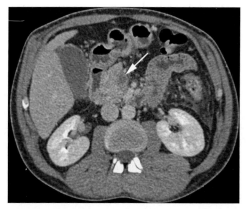

Fig. 10. Axial image shows thrombosis of the SMV (*arrow*). The proximal small bowel is also moderately thickened.

Even in the absence of symptoms, patients may have clinically significant disease. Up to 18% of patients over age 65 years have greater than 50% stenosis of a mesenteric artery, usually without symptoms [48,49]. Patients generally are asymptomatic until at least two of three major mesenteric vessels, typically the SMA and celiac artery, become severely stenotic or occluded (Fig. 13). Long-term studies have shown that as many as 86% of asymptomatic patients with greater than 50% stenosis of the mesenteric arteries eventually develop symptoms [50]. Mortality is approximately 40%.

Other causes of chronic mesenteric ischemia unrelated to atherosclerotic disease include vasculitis, fibromuscular dysplasia, median arcuate ligament syndrome, and tumor encasement. Radiation therapy can cause scarring and narrowing of the mesenteric vessels. Rarely, venous thrombosis or stenosis results in symptoms of chronic ischemia.

Symptoms of chronic mesenteric ischemia develop slowly over time, corresponding to a gradual reduction in blood flow to the intestines. Patients who have chronic mesenteric ischemia typically experience epigastric pain 15 to 60 minutes after a meal, as a result of increased demand for mesenteric blood flow [44]. The pain may last for several hours. Weight loss is common, a result of both pain and a change in dietary habits. Patients may even develop sitophobia, a fear of food or eating. Weight loss also may be caused by damage to the intestinal mucosa, with malabsorption of nutrients. Often patients experience symptoms for a year or more before seeking medical treatment.

Symptoms occur when collateral pathways no longer deliver an adequate supply of blood to the intestine (Fig. 14) [50]. The first of two major collateral pathways consists of the pancreaticoduodenal arteries, which connect the celiac axis and the SMA and permit both antegrade and retrograde blood flow, depending on the site of occlusion. The second set of major collateral pathways consists of the arc of Riolan and the marginal artery of Drummond, which allow communication between the SMA and IMA. In severe cases, compromise of the celiac axis, SMA, and IMA can result in the development of unusual collateral pathways composed of the pelvic, lumbar, or phrenic arteries [43].

Revascularization, either surgical or catheter-based, is the leading treatment for chronic mesenteric ischemia. Surgical bypass grafting, either retrograde or antegrade, usually involves the external iliac vessels. Transaortic endarterectomy is another surgical revascularization option. Regardless of the surgical approach, recurrence of mesenteric ischemia at 3 years is approximately 11% [51]. A study from the Mayo Clinic demonstrated 5-year graft patency rates of 90% with triple-vessel bypass grafting,

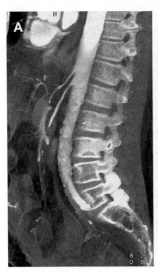
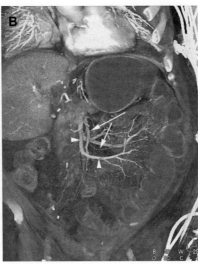

*Fig. 11.* (*A*) Sagittal volume-rendered 3D CTA in a patient who has hypotension and sepsis shows marked narrowing of the celiac axis and SMA. (*B*) Coronal oblique volume-rendered 3D CTA in the same patient shows pruning of the SMA branches (*arrows*). The mesenteric veins (*arrowheads*) are prominent. The small bowel is dilated and fluid filled.

54% with double-vessel bypass grafting, and 0% with single-vessel bypass grafting [52].

Percutaneous interventions include embolectomy, thrombolysis, angioplasty, and stenting [53,54]. Long-term data on percutaneous interventions are limited, but there is a growing trend in favor of percutaneous intervention as first-line therapy for chronic mesenteric ischemia. Some data suggest that percutaneous revascularization of only one stenotic mesenteric vessel may be sufficient to establish adequate blood flow to the

intestine, except in the case of high-grade stenoses (>70%).

### Diagnosis

Conventional invasive angiography is considered the criterion for the diagnosis of chronic mesenteric ischemia. There are other, less invasive ways to suggest the diagnosis, however. Duplex ultrasound, especially of the proximal arteries, can be used to measure blood flow before and after a meal. MR angiography also can be performed pre- and postprandially and is a safe option for patients who cannot tolerate iodinated contrast material. For most patients suspected of having chronic mesenteric ischemia, however, CT and CTA are the preferred noninvasive diagnostic studies.

In addition to being noninvasive, CTA offers a more complete examination than conventional angiography. CT angiographic images visualize distal vascular segments better, can be viewed in any projection, and depict vascular narrowing and also atherosclerotic plaque itself. In addition, CT enables evaluation of the bowel.

Stueckle and coworkers [55] evaluated 52 patients using both four-slice MDCT and conventional angiography. They found that CT accurately imaged the aorta and its branches, correctly diagnosing SMA stenosis in four patients and IMA occlusion in three.

Several CT findings are consistent with chronic mesenteric ischemia. Chief among them are calcified and noncalcified atherosclerotic plaque, typically in the celiac axis and SMA and less commonly in the IMA (Fig. 15). The atheroma usually is found in the proximal segment of the vessel, within a few centimeters of the origin [56].

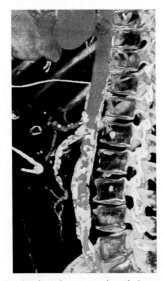

*Fig. 12.* Sagittal volume-rendered image demonstrates extensive calcified atherosclerotic plaque in the aorta and mesenteric arteries. Although significant plaque is present, there is no luminal narrowing. This patient has no signs or symptoms of ischemia.

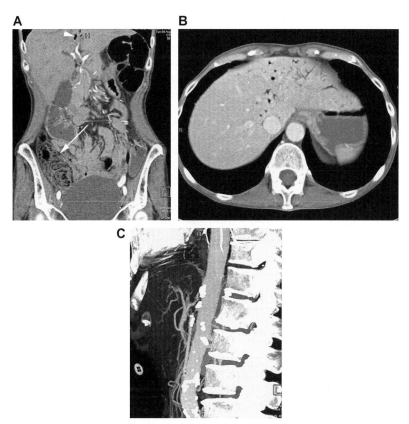

*Fig. 13.* (*A*) Coronal MPR in a patient with severe abdominal pain shows pneumatosis (*arrow*) in the right lower quadrant. Portal venous gas (*arrowhead*) is present also. (*B*) Axial image of the liver shows extensive portal venous air. (*C*) Sagittal volume-rendered 3D CTA shows extensive atherosclerosis of the celiac and SMA. At surgery the patient was found to have acute on cnronic ischemia. The infarcted bowel was resected, and a mesenteric bypass graft was placed.

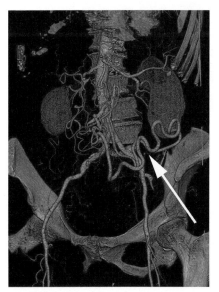

*Fig. 14.* Coronal volume-rendered 3D CTA in a patient who has chromic mesenteric ischemia shows a dilated collateral vessel (*arrow*) connecting the IMA and SMA.

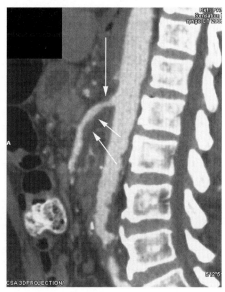

*Fig. 15.* Sagittal volume-rendered 3D CTA shows extensive atherosclerotic plaque (*arrows*) in a diabetic patient.

Focal narrowing is another common finding, with a stenosis of greater than 50% being considered hemodynamically significant. Diffuse atherosclerosis of a vessel is sometimes observed in patients who have advanced diabetes or severe renal disease. Such patients may develop ischemic symptoms in the absence of a critical stenosis, as a result of narrowing over a long segment of the vessel. Small, attenuated, pruned vessels are also common findings.

The presence of collateral pathways is a key diagnostic finding in chronic mesenteric ischemia. For example, prominent vessels around the head of the pancreas should raise immediate suspicion of a hemodynamically significant stenosis of the celiac axis resulting in dilatation of the pancreaticoduodenal arteries (Fig. 16).

## Summary

Technological advances in CT scanners and 3D computer workstations have, in general, improved

visualization of the bowel. CT angiography, in particular, enables visualization of the mesenteric vessels in remarkable detail. As a result, CT is becoming the preferred method for imaging the small intestine and mesenteric vessels in patients suspected of having acute or chronic mesenteric ischemic as well as other causes of acute abdominal pain.

MDCT of the mesenteric vessels and small intestine requires careful attention to the selection and delivery of oral and intravenous contrast material. Neutral contrast agents facilitate differentiation of the bowel wall and intraluminal contents and improve demonstration of mural features. Rapid injection of intravenous contrast material, in combination with a dual-phase image acquisition protocol, ensures excellent visualization of both the mesenteric arteries and the mesenteric veins.

The distal branches of mesenteric arteries measure 1 mm or less in diameter. It is critical, therefore, that the CT scan be performed using the thinnest possible collimation, typically 0.6 mm on a 64-slice scanner. The use of 0.75-mm

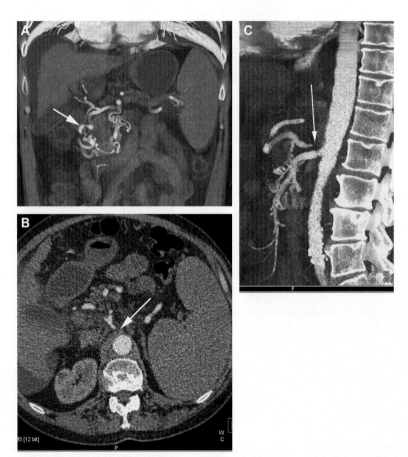

*Fig. 16.* (*A*) Coronal volume-rendered 3D CTA shows a dilated gastroduodenal artery (*arrow*). This is a common collateral pathway between the SMA and celiac. The patient also has cirrhosis, splenomegaly, and ascites. (*B*) Axial image in the same patient shows occlusion of the proximal celiac axis (*arrow*). (*C*) Sagittal volume-rendered 3D CTA nicely shows the occlusion of the proximal celiac axis (*arrow*) caused by atherosclerosis.

overlapping slices and a reconstruction interval of 0.5 mm produces a volume data set that is ideal for 3D image interpretation. A sagittal projection is most useful when evaluating the origin and proximal portions of the mesenteric arteries and fori-dentifying anatomic variants. A coronal or coronal oblique projection is preferred for detailed examination of branch vessels and for evaluation of the small intestine.

Key vascular findings in acute mesenteric ischemia include atheroma, embolism or thrombus, stenosis, and tumor encasement. In low-flow states or hypovolemia, CT demonstrates small, attenuated, pruned vessels. Air in the mesenteric vein, portal vein, or liver is a very late finding. The presence of collateral pathways is a key vascular finding in chronic mesenteric ischemia, particularly in a patient who has atherosclerotic plaque in the mesenteric vessels and a clinical history of gradually worsening postprandial pain. Key bowel findings suggestive of ischemia include thickening of the bowel wall, bowel dilatation, abnormal bowel wall attenuation, and an abnormal pattern of bowel wall enhancement.

Mesenteric ischemia, whether acute or chronic, is associated with a high mortality (70% and 40%, respectively). MDCT angiography has the potential to improve diagnosis and patient outcomes dramatically.

## References

[1] Horton KM, Eng J, Fishman EK. Normal enhancement of the small bowel: evaluation with spiral CT. J Comput Assist Tomogr 2000;24(1):67–71.

[2] Ramsay DW, Markham DH, Morgan B, et al. The use of dilute Calogen as a fat density oral contrast medium in upper abdominal computed tomography, compared with the use of water and positive oral contrast media. Clin Radiol 2001; 56(8):670–3.

[3] Malik N, Khandelwal N, Garg K, et al. Computed tomography of the abdomen with fat density oral contrast medium. Australas Radiol 1992; 36(1):31–3.

[4] Thompson SE, Raptopoulos V, Sheiman RL, et al. Abdominal helical CT: milk as a low-attenuation oral contrast agent. Radiology 1999;211(3):870–5.

[5] Pochaczevsky R. Carbon dioxide as a low-attenuation oral contrast agent. Radiology 2000; 214(3):918.

[6] Megibow AJ, Babb JS, Hecht EM, et al. Evaluation of bowel distention and bowel wall appearance by using neutral oral contrast agent for multidetector row CT. Radiology 2006;238(1):87–95.

[7] Lindner HH, Kemprud E. A clinicoanatomical study of the arcuate ligament of the diaphragm. Arch Surg 1971;103(5):600–5.

[8] Sproat IA, Pozniak MA, Kennell TW. US case of the day. Median arcuate ligament syndrome (celiac artery compression syndrome). Radiographics 1993;13(6):1400–2.

[9] Bron KM, Redman HC. Splanchnic artery stenosis and occlusion. Incidence; arteriographic and clinical manifestations. Radiology 1969;92(2): 323–8.

[10] Horton KM, Talamini MA, Fishman EK. Median arcuate ligament syndrome: evaluation with CT angiography. Radiographics 2005;25(5):1177–82.

[11] Szilagyi DE, Rian RL, Elliott JP, et al. The cardiac artery compression syndrome: does it exist? Surgery 1972;72(6):849–63.

[12] Stoney RJ, Cunningham CG. Acute mesenteric ischemia. Surgery 1993;114(3):489–90.

[13] Schneider TA, Longo WE, Ure T, et al. Mesenteric ischemia. Acute arterial syndromes. Dis Colon Rectum 1994;37(11):1163–74.

[14] Brandt LJ, Boley SJ. AGA technical review on intestinal ischemia. American Gastrointestinal Association. Gastroenterology 2000;118(5):954–68.

[15] Kirkpatrick ID, Kroeker MA, Greenberg HM. Biphasic CT with mesenteric CT angiography in the evaluation of acute mesenteric ischemia: initial experience. Radiology 2003;229(1): 91–8.

[16] Lee R, Tung HK, Tung PH, et al. CT in acute mesenteric ischaemia. Clin Radiol 2003;58(4): 279–87.

[17] Kim JY, Ha HK, Byun JY, et al. Intestinal infarction secondary to mesenteric venous thrombosis: CT-pathologic correlation. J Comput Assist Tomogr 1993;17(3):382–5.

[18] Alpern MB, Glazer GM, Francis IR. Ischemic or infarcted bowel: CT findings. Radiology 1988; 166(1 Pt 1):149–52.

[19] Wiesner W, Khurana B, Ji H, et al. CT of acute bowel ischemia. Radiology 2003;226(3):635–50.

[20] Clark RA. Computed tomography of bowel infarction. J Comput Assist Tomogr 1987;11(5): 757–62.

[21] Bartnicke BJ, Balfe DM. CT appearance of intestinal ischemia and intramural hemorrhage. Radiol Clin North Am 1994;32(5):845–60.

[22] Taourel PG, Deneuville M, Pradel JA, et al. Acute mesenteric ischemia: diagnosis with contrast-enhanced CT. Radiology 1996;199(3):632–6.

[23] Salzano A, De Rosa A, Carbone M, et al. Computerized tomography features of intestinal infarction: 56 surgically treated patients of which 5 with reversible mesenteric ischemia. Radiol Med (Torino) 1999;97(4):246–50 [in Italian].

[24] Kernagis LY, Levine MS, Jacobs JE. Pneumatosis intestinalis in patients with ischemia: correlation of CT findings with viability of the bowel. AJR Am J Roentgenol 2003;180(3):733–6.

[25] McKinsey JF, Gewertz BL. Acute mesenteric ischemia. Surg Clin North Am 1997;77(2):307–18.

[26] Kazmers A. Operative management of chronic mesenteric ischemia. Ann Vasc Surg 1998;12(3): 299–308.

[27] Bakal CW, Sprayregen S, Wolf EL. Radiology in intestinal ischemia. Angiographic diagnosis and management. Surg Clin North Am 1992;72(1): 125–41.

[28] Ha HK, Lee SH, Rha SE, et al. Radiologic features of vasculitis involving the gastrointestinal tract. Radiographics 2000;20(3):779–94.

[29] Levine SM, Hellmann DB, Stone JH. Gastrointestinal involvement in polyarteritis nodosa (1986–2000): presentation and outcomes in 24 patients. Am J Med 2002;1125:386–91.

[30] Siskind BN, Burrell MI, Pun H, et al. CT demonstration of gastrointestinal involvement in Henoch-Schonlein syndrome. Gastrointest Radiol 1985;10(4):352–4.

[31] Jeong YK, Ha HK, Yoon CH, et al. Gastrointestinal involvement in Henoch-Schonlein syndrome: CT findings. AJR Am J Roentgenol 1997; 168(4):965–8.

[32] Andrews PA, Frampton G, Cameron JS. Antiphospholipid syndrome and systemic lupus erythematosus. Lancet 1993;342(8877):988–9.

[33] Lalani TA, Kanne JP, Hatfield GA, et al. Imaging findings in systemic lupus erythematosus. Radiographics 2004;24(4):1069–86.

[34] Ha HK, Lee HJ, Yang SK, et al. Intestinal Behcet syndrome: CT features of patients with and patients without complications. Radiology 1998; 209(2):449–54.

[35] Corbetti F, Vigo M, Bulzacchi A, et al. CT diagnosis of spontaneous dissection of the superior mesenteric artery. J Comput Assist Tomogr 1989; 13(6):965–7.

[36] Messina LM, Shanley CJ. Visceral artery aneurysms. Surg Clin North Am 1997;77(2):425–42.

[37] Pilleul F, Beuf O. Diagnosis of splanchnic artery aneurysms and pseudoaneurysms with special reference to contrast enhanced 3D magnetic resonance angiography: a review. Acta Radiol 2004; 45(7):702–8.

[38] Rhee RY, Gloviczki P, Mendonca CT, et al. Mesenteric venous thrombosis: still a lethal disease in the 1990s. J Vasc Surg 1994;20(5):688–97.

[39] Sack J, Aldrete JS. Primary mesenteric venous thrombosis. Surg Gynecol Obstet 1982;154(2): 205–8.

[40] Martinez JP, Hogan GJ. Mesenteric ischemia. Emerg Med Clin North Am 2004;22(4):909–28.

[41] Newman TS, Magnuson TH, Ahrendt SA, et al. The changing face of mesenteric infarction. Am Surg 1998;64(7):611–6.

[42] Diamond SM, Emmett M, Henrich WL. Bowel infarction as a cause of death in dialysis patients. JAMA 1986;256(18):2545–7.

[43] Cognet F, Ben Salem D, Dranssart M, et al. Chronic mesenteric ischemia: imaging and percutaneous treatment. Radiographics 2002; 22(4):863–79 [discussion: 879–80].

[44] Cademartiri F, Raaijmakers RH, Kuiper JW, et al. Multi-detector row CT angiography in patients with abdominal angina. Radiographics 2004; 24(4):969–84.

[45] Moawad J, McKinsey JF, Wyble CW, et al. Current results of surgical therapy for chronic mesenteric ischemia. Arch Surg 1997;132(6):613–8 [discussion: 618–9].

[46] Derrick JR, Pollard HS, Moore RM. The pattern of arteriosclerotic narrowing of the celiac and superior mesenteric arteries. Ann Surg 1959;149(5): 684–9.

[47] Reiner L, Jimenez FA, Rodriguez FL. Atherosclerosis in the mesenteric circulation. Observations and correlations with aortic and coronary atherosclerosis. Am Heart J 1963;66:200–9.

[48] Rootbottom CA, Dubbins PA. Significant disease of the celiac and superior mesenteric arteries in asymptomatic patients: predictive value of Doppler sonography. AJR Am J Roentgenol 1993; 161(5):985–8.

[49] Thomas JH, Blake K, Pierce GE, et al. The clinical course of asymptomatic mesenteric arterial stenosis. J Vasc Surg 1998;27(5):840–4.

[50] Sreenarasimhaiah J. Chronic mesenteric ischemia. Best Pract Res Clin Gastroenterol 2005; 19(2):283–95.

[51] Park WM, Cherry KJ Jr, Chua HK, et al. Current results of open revascularization for chronic mesenteric ischemia: a standard for comparison. J Vasc Surg 2002;35(5):853–9.

[52] McAfee MK, Cherry KJ Jr, Naessens JM, et al. Influence of complete revascularization on chronic mesenteric ischemia. Am J Surg 1992;164(3): 220–4.

[53] Matsumoto AH, Angle JF, Spinosa DJ, et al. Percutaneous transluminal angioplasty and stenting in the treatment of chronic mesenteric ischemia: results and longterm followup. J Am Coll Surg 2002;194(1Suppl):S22–31.

[54] Maspes F, Mazzetti di Pietralata G, Gandini R, et al. Percutaneous transluminal angioplasty in the treatment of chronic mesenteric ischemia: results and 3 years of follow-up in 23 patients. Abdom Imaging 1998;23(4):358–63.

[55] Stueckle CA, Haegele KF, Jendreck M, et al. Multislice computed tomography angiography of the abdominal arteries: comparison between computed tomography angiography and digital subtraction angiography findings in 52 cases. Australas Radiol 2004;2(48):142–7.

[56] Jarvinen O, Laurikka J, Sisto T, et al. Atherosclerosis of the visceral arteries. Vasa 1995;24(1): 9–14.

RADIOLOGIC
CLINICS
OF NORTH AMERICA

Radiol Clin N Am 45 (2007) 289–301

ELSEVIER
SAUNDERS

# CT Enteroclysis: Techniques and Applications

Dean D.T. Maglinte, MD[a,*], Kumaresan Sandrasegaran, MD[a],
John C. Lappas, MD[b]

- Technical modifications
   *CT enteroclysis with neutral enteral
   and intravenous contrast*
   *CT enteroclysis with positive enteral
   contrast*
   *CT parameters*
- Clinical indications
- Miscellaneous applications

- Relevance of CT enteroclysis in the elective
   investigation of small bowel disease
   *Precapsule endoscopy*
   *Postcapsule endoscopy*
- Disadvantages and pitfalls of CT
   enteroclysis
- Summary
- References

Radiologic investigations have dominated small bowel imaging for the entire last century until the advent of capsule endoscopy [1]. Traditionally, the small bowel follow-through has been the most commonly performed method of examination because of its simplicity, availability, and low cost. Barium enteroclysis, however, has been shown to have higher overall accuracy and reliability at the expense of increased invasiveness and decreased patient tolerance without the use of conscious sedation [2,3]. The disadvantage of all fluoroscopic barium small bowel examinations is their inability to provide extraluminal information that may have important clinical implications for patients who have diseases of the small bowel. Much of the diagnostic information from barium studies was derived from the indirect mucosal and mural changes produced by lesions within or outside the lumen allowing substantial intra- and interobserver variation and difficulty in interpreting equivocal or

sometimes overt findings. This disadvantage has become particularly apparent with the increased use of contrast-enhanced CT studies [4–6]. A comparison of barium enteroclysis and abdominal CT performed on the same patients who had small bowel Crohn's disease demonstrated a much higher yield for CT in revealing mural and extraluminal manifestations of disease, including abscesses. Enteroclysis, however, was superior for diagnosing luminal abnormalities including bowel obstruction (especially low-grade), sinus tracts, fistulae, and ulcerations, mainly as a result of the enteral volume challenge generated by the controlled infusion of the contrast agent [7]. It was only a matter of time until CT enteroclysis (CTE) was developed to overcome the individual deficiencies of each method and to combine the advantages of both examinations into one technique.

Initially reported by Kloppel and colleagues in 1992 [8], CTE was shown to be highly accurate in

[a] Department of Radiology, Indiana University School of Medicine, 550 N. University Blvd, UH 0279, Indianapolis, IN 46202-5253, USA
[b] Department of Radiology, Wishard Memorial Hospital, Indiana University School of Medicine, 1001 West 10th Street, Indianapolis, IN 46202-5253, USA
* Corresponding author.
*E-mail address:* dmaglint@iupui.edu (D.D.T. Maglinte).

doi:10.1016/j.rcl.2007.03.008

depicting mucosal abnormalities as well as bowel thickening, fistulae, and other extraintestinal complications of Crohn's disease. The first North American study was performed in patients suspected of having small bowel obstruction [9]. Bender and colleagues [9] showed that CTE was superior to conventional CT for the diagnosis of lower grades of small bowel obstruction and also was able to reveal the nature of the obstructive lesion. Notably, in these patients, adhesions were inferred on conventional CT when no mass, inflammatory changes, or any other significant pathology was seen at the site of obstruction.

The mesenteric small intestine remains the most difficult segment of the intestinal tract to examine because of its length and overlapping position within the peritoneal cavity. Technologic advances have been clinically driven and have made small bowel imaging a rapidly changing field [10]. The limitations of commonly used methods of small bowel imaging to answer questions that are relevant to management of patients with suspected or known small bowel disease have led to refinements of previously used techniques and introduction of newer methods of examination. The introduction of multislice CT technology with its ability to scan larger volumes at a faster speed and the use of thinner section collimation allowing acquisition of near-isotropic or isotropic voxels has made high-resolution multiplanar reformatting a simple practical procedure with newer software [11–17]. This technology also has resulted in improved performance and feasibility of CTE and increased use of this method around the world [18–21].

At the same time, progress in endoscopy has been remarkable also. Capsule endoscopy and, recently, double-balloon enteroscopy have allowed full exploration of the small bowel. The latter technique is completed with interventional capabilities that previously were available only through intraoperative enteroscopy [22,23]. This article examines the techniques of CTE and presents an overview of its clinical applications relative to other methods of small bowel imaging.

## Technical modifications

When CTE was first reported, dilute positive enteral contrast was used. Since that time, two technical modifications have been adapted in the performance of CTE. One uses neutral enteral contrast with intravenous contrast enhancement, and the other uses positive enteral contrast [15–21]. Each modification is associated with technical differences that are described separately. For both modifications, bowel preparation includes a low-residue diet, ample fluids, a laxative used the day before the

examination, and nothing taken by mouth on the day of the examination. As with barium enteroclysis, patients are given the option of having conscious sedation when using a 13-F enteroclysis catheter (MEC Cook Inc. Bloomington IN) [13,15].

## CT enteroclysis with neutral enteral and intravenous contrast

Neutral enteral contrast agents that may be used for CTE include 0.5% methylcellulose, water, and dilute barium. Each neutral enteral contrast agent has distinct advantages and disadvantages, and all have been used successfully. Methylcellulose was used initially by some radiologists because of perceived slower absorption compared with water [18–21], but it is no longer commercially available in the United States. The authors currently use water or dilute barium. In comparison with oral administration of water, in which rapid absorption results in collapsed bowel, absorption is not as fast when water is infused into the small bowel. Water also is eliminated rapidly. Because of its low viscosity, water can be infused at a faster rate than other agents and with a decreased incidence of vomiting. Other advantages of water include its lower attenuation and cost. The lower attenuation of water compared with methylcellulose and dilute barium contrasts well with the mucosal enhancement produced by the intravenous contrast agent and allows a global look at all abdominal and pelvic organs (Fig. 1). In a busy tertiary care facility, performing an average of four CTE daily, the authors have not had a patient develop complications with the use of water. The speed of acquisition with multislice CT technology, the fast rate of enteral infusion used, the use of a hypotonic agent, and the volume infused keep the small intestine distended.

Dilute barium contains a flavoring agent and additives to decrease absorption and has a slightly higher attenuation than water. Dilute barium has been used successfully without complications and is preferred by the authors for the CT oral hyperhydration method (CT enterography, a non–enteral volume-challenged examination) [24]. Dilute barium also may have an advantage in staging Crohn's disease and in demonstrating sinus tracts or fistulae (Fig. 2).

The amount and rate of administration of intravenous contrast depends on the radiologist's individual preference. The authors prefer CT acquisition during the late arterial/early portal venous phase when maximum intestinal mucosal enhancement occurs [25] because it also allows evaluation of the intestinal vasa recta.

Because of the lack of viscosity of water and the low viscosity of the other neutral enteral agents, a small balloon catheter can be used (9 F Maglinte

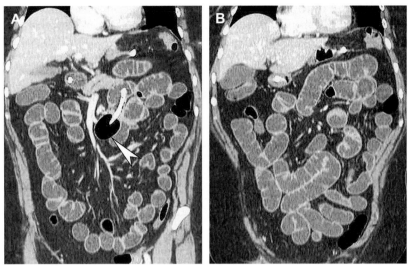

*Fig. 1.* CTE with neutral enteral (water) and intravenous contrast enhancement. (*A*) Enteroclysis balloon inflated with air (*arrowhead*) to the left of vertebra. Intestinal vascularity is imaged optimally in the late arterial phase, which is important in staging Crohn's disease and detecting neoplasms. Pancreatic parenchyma is well demonstrated in this phase of acquisition. (*B*) The lower viscosity of water allows faster infusion rates (100–150 mL/min) with reduced tendency of vomiting and uniform distention of the entire small intestine.

MiniCatheter, EZ EM Inc., Westbury, NY). This small, soft catheter may obviate the need for conscious sedation in many patients. The balloon and catheter tip ideally are positioned to the left of midline (Figs. 1A and 2B). In patients being evaluated for unexplained gastrointestinal bleeding or anemia, the balloon should be positioned in the proximal descending duodenum. The balloon is inflated with 30 to 40 mL of air. After balloon inflation, a 60-mL syringe of air is injected into the infusion lumen to determine if air refluxes proximal to the balloon. If necessary, additional air can be injected into the balloon to prevent reflux. This simple method decreases reflux of enteral contrast into the stomach and, in the authors' experience, decreases nausea and vomiting. Because neutral enteral contrast agents are not seen fluoroscopically, injection of air into the infusion lumen also allows the radiologist to see the location of the catheter tip in the bowel. This localization is important to prevent perforation from inadvertent catheter tip placement in a diverticulum. The authors'

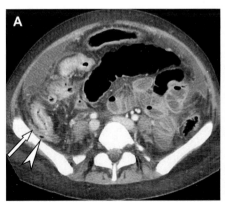
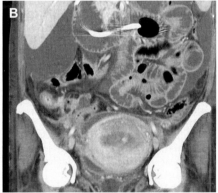

*Fig. 2.* CTE with dilute barium enteral contrast and intravenous contrast in the assessment of small bowel Crohn's disease. (*A*) Transverse image of 35-year-old woman who has a history of Crohn's disease, presenting with abdominal pain following an abortion 4 days earlier, showed extraluminal gas (*arrowhead*) adjacent to a loop of small bowel with mural thickening and increased attenuation compared with normal jejunal loops in left hemi-abdomen. The slightly increased attenuation of fluid (*arrow*) adjacent to the extraluminal gas indicated extravasation of dilute barium and allowed confident diagnosis of small bowel perforation from Crohn's disease. (*B*) Coronal image showed fluid around the uterus and in several peritoneal compartments. At surgery, a loculated abscess in the abdominal cavity from perforated small bowel Crohn's disease was confirmed.

technique for performing CTE with neutral enteral and intravenous contrast is summarized in Box 1.

In the fluoroscopic phase, the authors observe the position of the balloon and gauge the response of the patient to the rate of initial infusion (100 mL/min) after 500 mL is infused. The infusion rate is increased by 20 mL/min when dilute barium is used. If the balloon is pushed back to the descending duodenum at this rate, the authors re-advance the catheter tip and decrease the infusion rate to 80 mL/min. The authors also decrease the infusion rate to 80 mL/min iff patients, particularly those who have irritable bowel syndrome, complain of abdominal pain at this rate, even if the balloon is not pushed back. They raise the infusion rate by 10 mL/min from the initial rate (100 mL/min) on the CT table. If the patient evacuates some of the enteral contrast prematurely when no CT unit is immediately available, the authors infuse an additional liter on the CT table before giving intravenous contrast. Close coordination and cooperation between fluoroscopic and CT technologists has made premature evacuation of contrast a rare occurrence in the authors' practice. In patients who have had prior surgery involving the ileocecal valve, the authors decrease the amount infused at CT to about 1000 mL but increase the infusion rate to 130 mL/min if possible. The high rate of infusion keeps the small bowel distended longer. The spasmolytic agent (glucagon) keeps the small bowel aperistaltic and allows the patient to hold the large amount of contrast in the small bowel and colon. The authors give the glucagon intravenously in two small doses to diminish the nausea common with higher doses and to prolong its effect.

## CT enteroclysis with positive enteral contrast

Positive enteral contrast agents range from a 4% to 15% water-soluble contrast solution to dilute 6% barium solution [8,13]. The concentration used depends mostly on the radiologist's preference. The authors prefer an 11% iodine concentration of water-soluble contrast because this density allows diagnostic fluoroscopic observations as well as diagnostic radiographs. Assessment of subtle gradients from low-grade obstruction may be more apparent at fluoroscopy than with a single acquisition of CT images. Fluoroscopic evaluation with positive enteral contrast can help distinguish fixed (stenotic) segments of small bowel narrowing from spasm caused by active inflammation in patients who have Crohn's disease and can differentiate mild stenosis from normal peristaltic contractions. The changes in the caliber of the narrowing can be documented by real-time digital serial acquisition available with newer digital remote control fluoroscopic units.

Because infusion of positive enteral contrast is done under fluoroscopic control, the balloon and catheter tip can be positioned initially in the descending duodenum in patients who have a history of vomiting (Fig. 3). Otherwise, the catheter tip is advanced into the distal duodenum. Because of the viscosity of the contrast material used, the 13-F diagnostic enteroclysis or a 13.5-F catheter is used (MEC or MDEC, Cook, Inc., Bloomington, IN). After the balloon is inflated with 30 to 40 mL of air, contrast infusion is started. If, at the start of infusion with slower infusion rates (55–100 mL/min) the balloon is pushed back or contrast refluxes proximal to the balloon, the infusion is stopped, and the balloon is inflated further. Box 2 shows the authors' CTE protocol with positive enteral contrast.

Additional enteral contrast is infused on the CT table. If the patient prematurely eliminated contrast before CT acquisition, the amount used is gauged by how much the patient lost. The amount of enteral contrast also is decreased if an abnormality (mass or gradient) is seen in the jejunum fluoroscopically. Determination of the optimal infusion rate during the fluoroscopic phase is important when using positive enteral contrast, because the infusion rate is the main factor that keeps the small intestine distended during CT acquisition. Newer

---

**Box 1:  CT enteroclysis with neutral enteral and intravenous contrast**

*Fluoroscopic phase*
1. Position balloon in the proximal descending duodenum for evaluation of bleeding or anemia or in the distal duodenum to the left of the spine.
2. Give 0.3 mg glucagon intravenously.
3. Infuse 1.5 L of water or dilute barium at 100 mL/min; adjust rate as described in text.

Transfer patient to CT table.

*CT phase*
1. Give 0.3 mg glucagon intravenously.
2. Infuse 1.5 L of water or dilute barium at 100 mL/min. Give 2 L for large or tall patients, or when colon evaluation is important.
3. Administer intravenous contrast: rate = 4 mL/s; total volume = 150 mL.

Acquire CT at a 50-second delay
Deflate balloon and retract catheter to level of black marker (marker indicates tip of catheter is in the body of the stomach); decompress refluxed enteral contrast from stomach before withdrawing catheter.

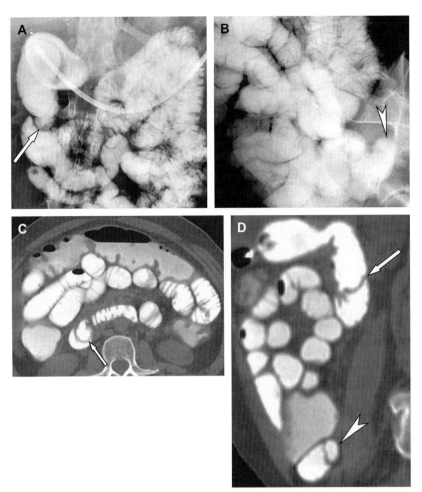

*Fig. 3.* CTE with positive enteral contrast in a middle-aged patient who had a history of postprandial vomiting. (*A*) Fluoroscopic phase. Note the position of the air-distended balloon in proximal duodenum. There was dilation of proximal descending duodenum above a curvilinear filling defect (*arrow*). This finding was confirmed subsequently at endoscopy as an intraluminal duodenal (windsock) diverticulum. (*B*) Spot oblique radiograph of pelvis showed an out-pouching from the antimesenteric margin (*arrowhead*) of a pelvic ileal loop indicating an incidental Meckel's diverticulum. (*C*) Transverse image at the level of the defect seen in panel A showed the same circumferential defect (*arrow*). (*D*) Sagittal reformation showed low-grade obstruction from the windsock diverticulum (*arrow*) and the incidental Meckel's diverticulum (*arrowhead*).

digital fluoroscopic units allow improved postprocessing of fluoroscopic images obtained during optimal distention and result in diagnostic single-contrast examinations when using an 11% solution of sodium diatrizoate. In some instances, subtle gradients of low-grade partial obstruction may be observed during the fluoroscopic phase but not on the CT images. The cause of the obstruction may not be seen fluoroscopically, however. When combined with the CT images, fluoroscopic observations recorded in on-the-spot radiographs add confidence to the diagnosis (see Fig. 3).

## CT parameters

Box 3 summarizes the CT parameters used at the authors' institution. Reformatted images are sent to the workstation for interpretation. The images obtained with the CT parameters used have less noise than when using isotropic voxels in the authors' patient population. Because of the large number of projection data images obtained when acquiring near-isotropic or isotropic voxels with multislice CT, practical handling of the source data or "smart postprocessing" is important to reduce the amount of data but at the same time increase the amount of information. This processing is tailored to the radiologist's needs. In the author's practice, interpretation is done on a separate workstation (Extended Brilliance Workspace, Philips Medical Imaging, Cleveland, OH) using interactive two-dimensional viewing (ie, viewing of axial, coronal, and sagittal images) with

**Box 2:** CT enteroclysis with positive enteral contrast

*Fluoroscopic phase*
1. Position balloon catheter tip in proximal descending duodenum or in distal duodenum if patient asthenic.
2. Infuse 11% water-soluble contrast at 55–150 mL/min (adjust rate for optimal enteral volume challenge as determined during fluoroscopy).
3. Infuse a total volume of 1 to 2 L, Stop when contrast is in the cecum. The amount of contrast needed to opacity pelvic small bowel loops using the adjusted rate of infusion at fluoroscopy is the amount infused at the CT table.
4. Limited fluoroscopy and radiography to cecum.

Transfer patient to CT.

*CT phase*
1. Infuse 500 mL to 1 L on CT table with infusion continued during scanning. The infusion rate is increased by 10 mL/min from the fluoroscopically determined infusion rate. Infuse volume as determined at fluoroscopy.
2. Withdraw enteroclysis catheter to stomach (black marker); suction refluxed contrast, then withdraw catheter.

**Box 3:** CT parameters using 16 and 64 multidetector channels

- Brilliance 16-Cchannel CT (MX 8000 IDT, Philips Medical Systems)

  Source: 16 × 1.5 mm
  Reformat: 2.0-mm slice width
  1.0-mm reconstruction interval

- Brilliance 40 or 64 (Philips Medical Systems)

  Source: 40 or 64 × 0.625 mm
  Reformat: 2.0-mm width
  1.0-mm reconstruction interval

Routine soft tissue viewing is used in CTE with neutral enteral and intravenous contrast (window width = 360 Houndsfield (H); window level = 40 H).
Small bowel windows (window width = 1200 H; window level = 200 H) are used for viewing positive enteral contrast CT [13]. The small bowel window settings used can be adjusted to individual preference (see Fig. 3C, D).

cross-referencing of abnormal or questionable findings. Selected significant reformatted images are sent to the picture archiving and communications system for the clinician's viewing.

## Clinical indications

The clinical applications of the two modifications of CTE overlap. In the authors' early experience, they performed CTE with positive enteral contrast for most investigations for possible small bowel obstruction (Fig. 4). Since the introduction of multislice CT technology, the authors use CTE with neutral enteral and intravenous contrast as their primary method of investigation when the scout

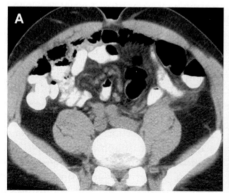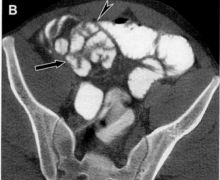

*Fig. 4.* A 38-year-old man with prior appendectomy presented with intermittent abdominal pain. (*A*) Conventional CT image showed no evidence of distended small bowel. (*B*) CTE with positive enteral contrast performed 3 days later showed distended proximal bowel loops with abrupt tapering of caliber (*arrowhead*) adjacent to the anterior parietal peritoneum. Distal small bowel contains enteral contrast but was nondistended (*arrow*). Low-grade obstruction was diagnosed and proven at laparoscopic examination as being caused by adhesions. (*From* Maglinte D. Essentials and clinical application of CT enteroclysis. In: Hodler J, Von Schulthess GK, Zollikofer Ch.L, editors. Diseases of the abdomen and pelvis. International Diagnostic Course in Davos syllabus. Milan: Springer-Verlag Italia; 2006; with permission.)

**Box 4:  Indications for CT enteroclysis with neutral enteral and intravenous contrast**

1. Unexplained gastrointestinal bleeding, or anemia when early Crohn's disease or nonsteroidal anti-inflammatory drug enteropathy is not a clinical consideration (Fig. 5)
2. Staging of known Crohn's disease (Fig. 6)
3. Unexplained abdominal pain with no evidence of significant small bowel distention on plain-film radiographs (Fig. 7)
4. Alternate examination before or after capsule endoscopy or when carbon dioxide double-contrast barium enteroclysis is not technically possible

Box 4 summarizes the authors' current clinical indications of CTE with neutral enteral and intravenous contrast. Box 5 summarizes their current clinical indications of CTE with positive enteral contrast.

## Miscellaneous applications

CTE has been of value in resolving the false-positive and false-negative interpretations from non–enteral volume-challenged small bowel studies that arise because of small bowel nonfilling, poor distention, and simulation of wall thickening or pseudodefect caused by retained fluid with positive oral contrast (see Fig. 8) [28]. In patients who have symptoms of proximal small bowel obstruction, the performance of CTE with the catheter tip in the descending duodenum has resulted in a more precise diagnosis (see Fig. 3).

Because of the high infusion rates used with CTE, the authors have reproduced abdominal pain and nausea in patients who have irritable bowel syndrome, and this finding may be important clinical information once organic disease is excluded [13]. Prompt adjustment of the infusion rate can

radiograph indicates small bowel is not distended, there is no contraindication to the use of intravenous iodinated contrast, and the patient has no history of vomiting. This modification is faster, reproducible, and allows a more global detailed evaluation of the small intestine and the entire abdomen. It is well tolerated by patients when simple technical guidelines are observed and uses less radiation than positive enteral contrast CTE.

**Box 5:  Indications for positive enteral contrast CT enteroclysis**

1. Suspected recurrent small bowel obstruction with vomiting or unexplained abdominal pain with negative or equivocal fluoroscopic or conventional CT examinations, or if intravenous contrast is contraindicated (Fig. 8)
2. Suspected small bowel disease (unexplained lower gastrointestinal bleeding, anemia, diarrhea, and history of nonsteroidal anti-inflammatory drug intake) and when intravenous contrast is contraindicated or air (carbon dioxide)–barium enteroclysis is not technically possible
3. Subsets of patients who have small bowel obstruction for whom general surgeons prefer conservative management and whose small bowel is distended on conventional abdominal radiography [26].

   a. Small bowel obstruction in the immediate postoperative period (Fig. 9)
   b. History of prior abdominal surgery for malignant tumor
   c. History of prior radiation therapy
   d. Crohn's disease with prior surgery.

The long decompression/enteroclysis catheter (MEC, Cook Inc. Bloomington, IN) (Fig. 9A) is used when the small bowl is distended and preliminary decompression is done [27].

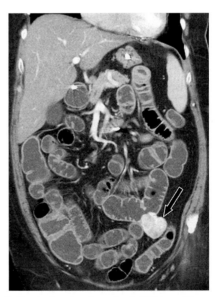

*Fig. 5.* Neutral enteral contrast CTE in a 63-year-old woman who had unexplained gastrointestinal bleeding. Capsule endoscopy demonstrated jejunal angioectasia but no mass (image not shown). CTE showed a 3-cm hypervascular submucosal mass (*arrow*) arising from the mid small bowel, proven to be a gastrointestinal stromal tumor at surgery. (*From* Maglinte D. Essentials and clinical application of CT enteroclysis. In: Hodler J, Von Schulthess GK, Zollikofer Ch.L, editors. Diseases of the abdomen and pelvis. International Diagnostic Course in Davos syllabus. Milan: Springer-Verlag Italia; 2006; with permission.)

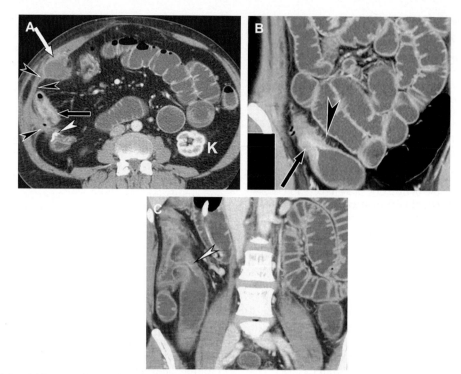

**Fig. 6.** (*A*) Axial image of neutral enteral contrast CTE in a 62-year-old woman who had Crohn's disease showed a long fistulous track (*black arrowheads*) extending from the inflamed cecum (*black arrow*) to an abscess (*white arrowhead*). Note the late arterial phase of intravenous contrast bolus, indicated by enhancement of left renal cortex (*K*). (*From* Maglinte D. Essentials and clinical application of CT enteroclysis. In: Hodler J, Von Schulthess GK, Zollikofer Ch.L, editors. Diseases of the abdomen and pelvis. International Diagnostic Course in Davos syllabus. Milan: Springer-Verlag Italia; 2006; with permission.) (*B*) Coronal reformation in a 59-year-old woman who had obstructive symptoms showed mural thickening (*arrow*) and prominent vasa recta (*arrowhead*). Note mucosal hyperenhancement and dilatation of the loop proximally suggesting small bowel obstruction from active inflammatory disease. (*C*) Coronal reformation of CTE in a 49-year-old woman who had known Crohn's disease and presented with symptoms of small bowel obstruction showed mild dilatation of distal ileum secondary to luminal narrowing of terminal ileum (*arrowhead*). Mural thickening has similar attenuation as soft tissue and lacks prominence of vasa recta, suggesting low-grade obstruction from fibrostenosing Crohn's disease.

diminish discomfort when it occurs. Because neutral enteral contrast is not seen fluoroscopically, CTE with this method is subject to difficulty in evaluating nondistended small bowel when patients vomit or inadvertently lose contrast per rectum (Fig. 10). Experience, adherence to technical details, and the proper selection of the method of CTE to be used for the clinical indication will result in a diagnostic examination.

## Relevance of CT enteroclysis in the elective investigation of small bowel disease

### Precapsule endoscopy

Except for the emergent clinical investigation for possible small bowel diseases, in which abdominal CT will remain the primary method of investigation, the role of imaging is likely to undergo reassessment based on results of capsule endoscopy in

the elective work-up of patients suspected of having small bowel disease [1]. In the patient who is not at risk for a potentially obstructing small bowel lesion, radiology may have a limited role. As stated earlier, when the indication raises the possibility of early Crohn's disease or nonsteroidal anti-inflammatory drug enteropathy, air double-contrast enteroclysis is the most reliable method of imaging. Air double-contrast barium enteroclysis seems to be the most sensitive method of radiologic investigation for the demonstration of the aphthoid lesions of early Crohn's disease (Fig. 11), erosions of nonsteroidal anti-inflammatory drug enteropathy, and characterizing a nonspecific stenosis [1]. Otherwise CTE should suffice for all precapsule radiologic investigations when there is the possibility of a potentially obstructing small bowel abnormality. There has been no report of capsule retention when enteroclysis was used to screen for possible strictures

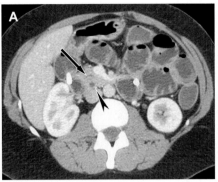
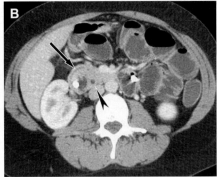

*Fig. 7.* A 40-year-old woman who had unexplained abdominal pain had CTE with neutral enteral and intravenous contrast enhancement. (*A*) Transverse image of upper abdomen showed normal proximal small bowel. Prominent pancreatic duct (*arrow*) coursed anterior to and did not join the common bile duct (*arrowhead*) in the major papilla indicating divisum anatomy. (*B*) Transverse image below the image shown in panel A showed pancreatic duct encircling duodenal lumen (*arrow*) indicating annular pancreas. Note distal common bile duct (*arrowhead*). Patient underwent duodenoduodenostomy for annular pancreas.

before capsule examination [29]. How the introduction of the patency capsule will affect the use of radiologic investigation remains to be seen [1].

## Postcapsule endoscopy

As with all examinations in which the human factor is involved, perceptive errors are inevitable.

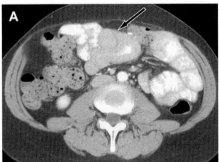
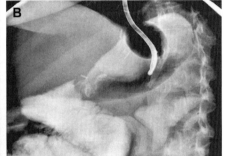
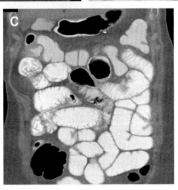

*Fig. 8.* A 75-year-old man with multiple prior upper abdominal surgeries, nausea and vomiting, and an abnormal conventional CT. (*A*) Transverse upper abdominal CT image showed thickened bowel loop with distorted lumen suspicious of a mass (*arrow*). (*B*) Patient subsequently underwent CTE with positive enteral constant. Fluoroscopic oblique radiograph following inflation of balloon distal to gastroesophageal junction showed Billroth I anatomy. Catheter and balloon are retracted at enteroclysis to prevent gastro-esophageal reflux during infusion in patients who have gastrojejunostomy or gastroduodenostomy. Note dilated jejunum. There was slow transit, but no mechanical obstruction or mass was seen during contrast infusion. (*C*) Coronal reformation of CTE showed mildly dilated proximal small bowel without evidence of mass. The pseudomass seen in panel A was probably caused by dysmotility from prior surgery.

The clinical significance of the diminutive red spots without positive evidence of bleeding and the superficial mucosal "scratches" shown by capsule endoscopy are increasingly being questioned [1]. A mucosal "scratch" is nonspecific and in some instances requires further characterization to make a precise diagnosis. Unpublished data in the authors' practice when an air double-contrast barium enteroclysis was done following capsule endoscopy interpreted by experienced endoscopists to assess extent or characterize Crohn's disease have shown limitations of capsule endoscopy in characterizing superficial ulcers and their precise location [1,30]. In one instance,

radiologic examination showed a giant Meckel's diverticulum with ulcerations in the junction of the diverticulum to the ileum. In another patient, nonsteroidal anti-inflammatory drug ulcers and diaphragm disease were shown by air enteroclysis but were ascribed by capsule endoscopy to Crohn's disease. The patient who has persistent symptoms or bleeding with negative capsule endoscopy requires accurate radiologic investigations (see Figs. 5 and 11). The authors have diagnosed a Meckel's diverticulum in a patient who had had a prior negative capsule endoscopy. Nonsteroidal anti-inflammatory drug ulcers were shown by air double-contrast barium enteroclysis. CTE with

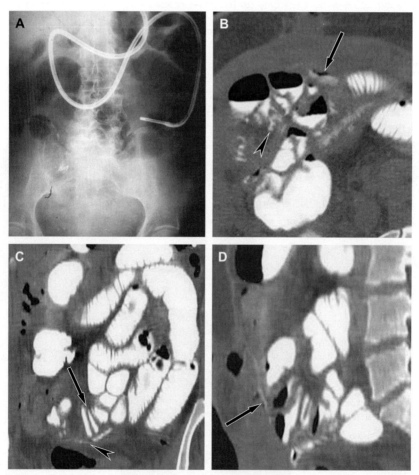

*Fig. 9.* Diagnosis and treatment of partial small bowel obstruction in immediate postoperative phase, using a decompression enteroclysis catheter in a 75-year-old woman who had had pelvic surgery 3 weeks earlier. (*A*) Conventional abdominal radiograph with tip of decompression/enteroclysis in proximal jejunum. Note that small bowel loops are distended. The tube was left in situ overnight for decompression. (*B*) Transverse image of lower abdomen following next-day infusion of positive enteral contrast showed dense anterior entero-parietal peritoneal (*arrow*) and entero-enteric (*arrowhead*) adhesions. (*C*) Coronal reformation of anterior abdomen showed dense adhesions (*arrow*) and a linear tract of contrast in the abdominal wall (*arrowhead*). (*D*) Sagittal reformation at midline showed dense adhesions and a small fistulous tract (*arrow*) at incision site. The triple lumen nasojejunal tube was left in place after enteroclysis for continued enteric decompression, with relief of obstructive symptoms. The fistula was corrected subsequently, but the patient did not need emergent reoperation.

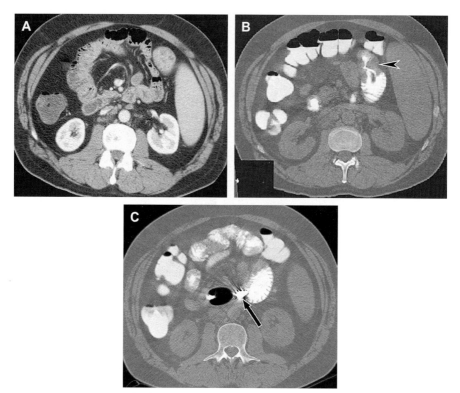

*Fig. 10.* A 48-year-old man presented with vomiting and weight loss. (*A*) During CTE with neutral enteral and intravenous contrast, the patient vomited, and the study was read as normal. Capsule endoscopy was unsuccessful because the capsule was retained. (*B, C*) Subsequent CTE with positive enteral contrast showed an annular obstructing mass (*arrowhead* in panel *B*) in the proximal jejunum and the retained capsule (*arrow* in panel *C*). The mass was proven to be adenocarcinoma. (*From* Maglinte D. Essentials and clinical application of CT enteroclysis. In: Hodler J, Von Schulthess GK, Zollikofer Ch.L, editors. Diseases of the abdomen and pelvis. International Diagnostic Course in Davos syllabus. Milan: Springer-Verlag Italia; 2006; with permission.)

neutral enteral and intravenous contrast is appropriate to assess further a possible submucosal mass found on capsule endoscopy.

## Disadvantages and pitfalls of CT enteroclysis

CTE requires placement of a nasoenteric tube for enteral contrast infusion. The associated discomfort may be alleviated by the use of conscious sedation and the use of smaller tubes [15]. Conscious sedation, however, requires dedicated personnel and makes the procedure longer and more expensive. In small institutions and non–tertiary care facilities, this procedure may not be practical. In patients who require nasogastric suction and potentially need a small bowel examination, the initial use of a decompression/enteroclysis catheter circumvents this disadvantage [27].

The logistics of performing CTE when the fluoroscopic suite is far from the CT area is a deterrent. The addition of CT to enteroclysis increases the cost of the procedure and the radiation exposure to patients

and radiologic personnel. CTE therefore should be done only when clinically indicated. Fluoroscopy should be limited when using positive enteral contrast CTE. CTE with neutral enteral and intravenous contrast should be used whenever feasible.

Radiation doses related to CTE remain a significant issue. The use of multidetector CT with 40 or more channels can reduce radiation by 10% to 66% because of more efficient detector configuration, automatic exposure controls, improved filters, and image postprocessing algorithms [31]. MR enteroclysis has the advantages of lack of radiation exposure and safer intravenous contrast agents but seems to be less accurate than CTE. In a prospective comparison of MR enteroclysis and CTE, the latter showed greater sensitivity and interobserver agreement for an array of pathologic signs of small bowel diseases [32].

## Summary

The early diagnosis of small bowel diseases will remain a diagnostic challenge to radiologists [33].

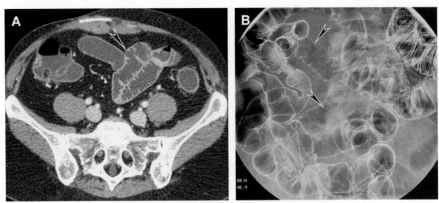

*Fig. 11.* A 49-year-old with unexplained iron deficiency anemia. Neutral enteral contrast CTE with (*A*) intravenous contrast and (*B*) air double-contrast barium enteroclysis performed within 2 weeks of each other showed a normal small bowel at CTE (*A, arrowhead*). On air double-contrast barium enteroclysis, multiple aphthae (*B, arrowheads*) were identified in the distal ileum, consistent with early Crohn's disease. The terminal ileum was unremarkable. Small ulcers are seen better with high-quality fluoroscopic air double-contrast barium enteroclysis than with CTE. Capsule endoscopy was negative. (*From* Maglinte D. Essentials and clinical application of CT enteroclysis. In: Hodler J, Von Schulthess GK, Zollikofer Ch.L, editors. Diseases of the abdomen and pelvis. International Diagnostic Course in Davos syllabus. Milan: Springer-Verlag Italia; 2006; with permission.)

CTE combines the advantages of CT and barium enteroclysis into one method of examination. Although it has disadvantages, the authors' and others' experience has shown its value in the investigation of small bowel diseases and in providing additional information relevant to the management of patients that was not obtained adequately by non–enteral volume-challenged small bowel examinations. The use of multislice technology and two-dimensional reformatting have made organs that are longer than wide, such as the mesenteric small intestine, easier to examine with CTE. In the nonemergent investigation of small bowel diseases CTE uses a hybrid imaging technique with a high negative predictive value and high sensitivity and specificity, a method of investigation needed in evaluating an organ such as the mesenteric small intestine with a low prevalence of disease whose clinical symptoms are nonspecific and mimicked by diseases of other abdominal organs. CTE is a reproducible method of small bowel examination. Its clinical application has been made more reliable and simpler to perform with multislice CT technology. CTE will keep radiology competitive in this era of high technology.

## References

[1] Maglinte D. Capsule imaging and the role of radiology in the investigation of diseases of the small bowel. Radiology 2005;236:763–7.
[2] Maglinte DD, Lappas JC, Kelvin FM, et al. Small bowel radiography: how, when, and why? Radiology 1987;163:197–305.
[3] Maglinte DD, Kelvin F, O'Connor K, et al. Current status of small bowel radiography. Abdom Imaging 1996;2:247–57.
[4] Buckley JA, Jones B, Fishman EK. Small bowel cancer: imaging features and staging. Radiol Clin North Am 1997;35:381–402.
[5] Fishman EK, Wolf EJ, Jones B, et al. CT evaluation of Crohn's disease: effect on patient management. AJR Am J Roentgenol 1987;148:537–40.
[6] Merine D, Fishman EK, Jones B. CT of the small bowel and mesentery. Radiol Clin North Am 1989;27:707–15.
[7] Maglinte DD, Hallett R, Rex D, et al. Imaging of small bowel Crohn's disease: can abdominal CT replace barium radiography? Emerg Radiol 2001; 8:127–33.
[8] Kloppel R, Thiele J, Bosse J. The Sellink CT method. Rofo 1992;156:291–2 [in German].
[9] Bender GN, Timmons JH, Williard WC, et al. Computed tomographic enteroclysis: one methodology. Invest Radiol 1996;31:43–9.
[10] Maglinte D. Small bowel imaging: a rapidly changing field and a challenge to radiology. Eur Radiol 2006;16:967–71.
[11] Caoili EM, Paulson EK. CT of small-bowel obstruction: another perspective using multiplanar reformations. AJR Am J Roentgenol 2000;174: 993–8.
[12] Ros PR, Ji H. CT: applications in the abdomen. Radiographics 2002;22:697–700.
[13] Maglinte DD, Bender GN, Heitkamp DE, et al. Multidetector-row helical CT enteroclysis. Radiol Clin North Am 2003;41(2):249–62.
[14] Horton KM, Fishman EK. The current status of multidetector row CT and three-dimensional imaging of the small bowel. Radiol Clin North Am 2003;41(2):199–212.

[15] Maglinte DD, Lappas JC, Heitkamp DE, et al. Technical refinements in enteroclysis. Radiol Clin North Am 2003;41:213–29.

[16] Gollub MS. Multidetector computed tomography enteroclysis of patients with small bowel obstruction: a volume rendered "surgical perspective". J Comput Assist Tomogr 2005;29:401–7.

[17] Maglinte DDT, Sandrasegaran K, Tann M. Advances in alimentary tract imaging. World J Gastroenterol 2006;12(20):3139–8145.

[18] Schober E, Turetschek K, Sschima W, et al. Methylcellulose enteroclysis spiral CT in the preoperative assessment of Crohn's disease: radiologic pathologic correlation [abstract]. Radiology 1997;205:717.

[19] Schoepf UJ, Holzknecht N, Matz C, et al. New developments in imaging the small bowel mutlislice computed tomography and negative contrast medium. In: Reiser MF, editor. Multislice CT. Berlin: Springer; 1997. p. 49–60.

[20] Rollandi GA, Curone PF, Conzi R, et al. Spiral CT of the abdomen alter distention of small bowel loops with transparent enema in patients with Crohn's disease. Abdom Imaging 1999;24(6):544–9.

[21] Romano S, De Lutio E, Rollandi GA, et al. Multidetector computed tomography enteroclysis (MDCT-E) with neutral enteral and intravenous contrast enhancement in tumor detection. Eur Radiol 2005;15:1178–83.

[22] Iddan GI, Swain CP. History and development of capsule endoscopy. Gastrointest Endosc Clin N Am 2004;14:1–9.

[23] Yamamoto H. Double balloon endoscopy. Clin Gastroenterol Hepatol 2005;3(7 Suppl 1):S27–9.

[24] Megibow AJ, Babb JS, Hecht EM, et al. Evaluation of bowel distention and bowel wall appearance by using neutral oral contrast agent for multidetector row CT. Radiology 2006;238(1):87–95.

[25] Horton KM, Eng J, Fishman EK. Normal enhancement of the small bowel: evaluation with spiral CT. J Comput Assist Tomogr 2000;24:67–71.

[26] Maglinte DDT, Kelvin FM, Sandrasegaran K, et al. Radiology of small bowel obstruction: contemporary approach and controversies. Abdom Imaging 2005;30:160–78.

[27] Maglinte D, Kelvin F, Rowe M, et al. Small-bowel obstruction: optimizing radiologic investigation and nonsurgical management. Radiology 2001;218:39–46.

[28] Maglinte DDT, Rhea JT, Ledbetter MS. The role of CT in acute abdominal disease: pitfalls and their lessons. In: Mann FA, editor. Emergency radiology: RSNA categorical course in diagnostic radiology 2004 syllabus. Oak Brook (IL): Radiologic Society of North America; 2004. p. 119–31.

[29] Voderholzer WA, Beinhoelz J, Rogalla P, et al. Small bowel involvement in Crohn's disease: a prospective comparison of wireless capsule endoscopy and computed tomography enteroclysis. Gut 2005;54:369–73.

[30] Maglinte DD. Invited commentary to: Hara AK, Leighton JA, Virender K, et al. Imaging of small bowel disease: comparison of capsule endoscopy, standard endoscopy, barium examination, and CT. Radiographics 2005;25:697–718.

[31] Mannudeep K, Rizzo SMR, Novelline RA. Technologic innovations in computer tomography dose reduction: implications in emergency settings. Emergency Radiology 2005;11:127–8.

[32] Duvoisin B, Meuli R, Michetti P, et al. Prospective comparison of MR enteroclysis with multidetector spiral-CT enteroclysis: interobserver agreement and sensitivity by means of "sign-by-sign" correlation. Eur Radiol 2003;13:1303–11.

[33] Maglinte D. The challenge to fluoroscopy in small bowel imaging in the 21st century. Presented at the European Society of Abdominal and Gastrointestinal Radiology/Society of Gastrointestinal Radiologists annual meeting and postgraduate course. Crete (Greece), June 20, 2006.

ELSEVIER
SAUNDERS

RADIOLOGIC
CLINICS
OF NORTH AMERICA

Radiol Clin N Am 45 (2007) 303–315

# CT Enterography: Noninvasive Evaluation of Crohn's Disease and Obscure Gastrointestinal Bleed

Scott R. Paulsen, MD[a], James E. Huprich, MD[a], Amy K. Hara, MD[b],*

Small bowel imaging is complicated by the length of the small bowel and overlapping loops. Cross-sectional imaging of the small bowel offers distinct advantages over fluoroscopic barium examination including depiction of the entire bowel wall and availability of multiplanar imaging. These tools prevent obscuration of small bowel loops by superimposition and also provide superior detection of abscesses and fistulas [1,2].

Although CT has been used previously to evaluate Crohn's disease (CD), the recent introduction of neutral oral contrast agents with improved luminal distention and advances in CT technology have converged to provide a new CT imaging technique specific for the small bowel known as CT enterography (CTE). CTE combines neutral or low-density oral contrast agents with intravenous contrast to depict small bowel diseases optimally. With this technique, small bowel vascular malformations, tumors, and inflammatory bowel diseases have all been detected [3].

This article describes the CTE technique and its specific application in the evaluation of CD and obscure gastrointestinal bleeding (OGIB).

## CT enterography technique

### Patient preparation

Patients are asked to abstain from any food or drink for 4 hours before scanning, which is identical to the authors' routine CT protocol using intravenous contrast.

Immediately before scanning patients ingest a neutral or low-density oral contrast agent such as water [4,5], water and methylcellulose [6], lactulose [7], or polyethylene glycol [3]. Although water is cheap and well tolerated, it often is absorbed too rapidly in fasting patients who have the poorest distention in the distal small bowel, the most common area of CD.

[a] Department of Diagnostic Radiology, Mayo Clinic Rochester, 200 First St. SW, Rochester, MN 55905, USA
[b] Department of Diagnostic Radiology, Mayo Clinic Arizona, 13400 East Shea Blvd, Scottsdale, AZ 85259, USA
* Corresponding author.
*E-mail address:* hara.amy@mayo.edu (A.K. Hara).

doi:10.1016/j.rcl.2007.03.009

The neutral oral contrast of choice for most CTE examinations is a low-concentration (0.1% weight of solute per volume of solution [w/v]) barium solution mixed with sorbitol. The sorbitol minimizes small bowel resorption of water and thereby improves luminal distention. The attenuation of the barium solution is 20 Hounsfield units (HU), and it is minimally hyperdense compared with water at CT. A recent study found that this low-concentration barium with sorbitol solution provided significantly better gastric and small bowel distention and visualization of mural features than an equal volume of water mixed with methylcellulose [6]. Low-concentration barium with sorbitol has also been shown to distend the bowel better than water [8,9] and with fewer side effects than polyethylene glycol [10].

Table 1 summarizes several different protocols for CTE. The amount and timing of oral contrast at CTE is not yet standardized. Studies have used 900 to 1800 mL given over time spans ranging from 30 minutes to 2 hours before CT. One study using 1200 mL of barium solution given over 30 minutes (900 mL over 20 minutes; 300 mL on the table) found that ileal distention was less than that of the duodenum and jejunum based on actual cross-sectional measurements of the best-distended loops, although radiologists did not detect any noticeable difference in bowel distention between the three segments [6]. Others prefer to give more barium solution (1800 mL) over a longer period of time (75 minutes) [11]. A multitude of factors that can affect the results make a comparison of different timing protocols difficult. These factors include (1) small bowel transit time, (2) scan delays (difficult intravenous access, or the scanner or patient running late), and (3) patient compliance with oral contrast ingestion. The authors have found that 1350 mL of barium solution given over 45 to 60 minutes provides excellent small bowel distention, with distention diminishing past 60 minutes.

In addition to oral contrast, several investigators have used other methods, such as glucagon (1 mg given intravenously or intramuscularly) and oral metoclopramide (10 mg), to improve small bowel distention [4,6,12]. No studies, however, have been reported to determine the usefulness of these agents for small bowel distention.

## Scanning techniques

### Intravenous contrast

For single-phase imaging at CTE, 150 mL of iohexol is administered at a rate of 4 mL/s. Although any multidetector scanner from 4 to 64 rows can perform the axial acquisition adequately, image quality of coronal reformatted images is best with the higher-performance scanners that can acquire at submillimeter collimation. The axial images are viewed at a 2- to 3.0-mm slice thickness with reconstruction interval of 1 to 1.5 mm. Coronal images are viewed at 2- to 3-mm slice thickness every 2 to 3 mm. Intravenous contrast amounts and radiation dose may be altered depending on patient size.

### Single-phase imaging technique

Single-phase imaging at CTE is done in most cases, particularly in the evaluation of CD and obstruction. The "enteric" phase is considered to be with a scan delay around 45 seconds, and many CTE protocols initiate scanning at this time. This timing is supported by a study in normal small bowel that showed slightly increased enhancement during the arterial phase (30 seconds) compared with the venous phase (60 seconds), although this difference was not thought to be clinically important [13]. The use of single-phase imaging in patients who have CD is supported also by another study that found no important differences between the arterial and venous phase images [4].

### Multiphasic imaging technique

Recently a multiphasic CTE protocol has been introduced for the evaluation of OGIB [11]. Because if the requirement for rapid, multiphase imaging, this technique is performed best on a 64-row detector scanner. Enteric and intravenous contrast

*Table 1:* **Comparison of oral contrast protocols for CT enterography**

| First author | Low-concentration barium with sorbitol solution | Other oral contrast | Amount (cm³) | Drinking time (min) |
|---|---|---|---|---|
| Huprich [11] | + | | 1800 | 75 |
| Al-Hawary [9] | + | Water | 1350 | 60 |
| Megibow [6] | + | Water + methycellulose | 1200 | 30 |
| Oliva [8] | + | Water, 2.1% barium sulfate | 900 | 60 |
| Bodily [5] | | Water | 1800 | 75 |
| Columbel [12] | | Water + methycellulose | 1500 | 75 |
| Hara [33] | | Water | 1500 | 45 |

administration are the same as for single-phase CTE. With this protocol, no precontrast images are obtained. Bolus triggering is performed by placing an region of interest (ROI) cursor over the descending aorta 2 cm above the diaphragm. The ROI trigger threshold is set at 150 HU, with scanning initiated 6 seconds later. Scanning is performed from the diaphragm to the symphysis pubis during each of three phases: (1) a bolus-triggered arterial phase, (2) at 20 to 25 seconds (enteric phase), and (3) at 70 to 75 seconds (delayed phase) after the beginning of the arterial phase acquisition.

Axial images are reconstructed at 2-mm slice width and 1-mm interval. Coronal images are reconstructed from the retroperitoneal border to the anterior abdominal wall at 2-mm slice width and 1-mm interval.

## Imaging findings

### Differences in bowel appearance using neutral versus positive oral contrast

The use of neutral oral contrast in conjunction with intravenous contrast juxtaposes enhancing mucosa with the fluid-attenuating luminal contents (Fig. 1A) [14] and thereby facilitates detection of subtle mucosal enhancement [4,15]. Positive oral contrast agents actually may obscure pathologically enhancing mucosa (Fig. 1B) because of the lack of difference in attenuation between enhancing mucosa and luminal contents [3]. Bowel wall thickness

can be assessed using positive or negative oral contrast.

## Crohn's disease

### Disease distribution

CD is recognizable as discontinuous, segmental, often multifocal inflammation that may affect any part of the gastrointestinal tract from mouth to anus. Involvement of the GI tract proximal to the jejunum, however, is rare and when present is almost always in association with involvement of the lower gastrointestinal tract. Most commonly, in nearly half of patients, CD is seen in both the small and large bowel. In approximately one third of patients, inflammation is isolated to the small bowel (mostly in the terminal ileum). Inflammation is confined to the colon in up to 20% of patients [16].

### Enteric findings

The classic CT imaging features of active small bowel CD are bowel wall thickening, mural hyperenhancement, and mural stratification. Chronic changes of CD include strictures and submucosal fatty deposition in the bowel wall.

Small bowel wall thickening has been shown to be a highly sensitive and specific finding of active CD [5,17–19]. Typically, small bowel mural thickness of greater than 3 mm is considered pathologic. Some studies have suggested that the thickness of the bowel wall correlates with disease activity, so that markedly thickened segments indicate active

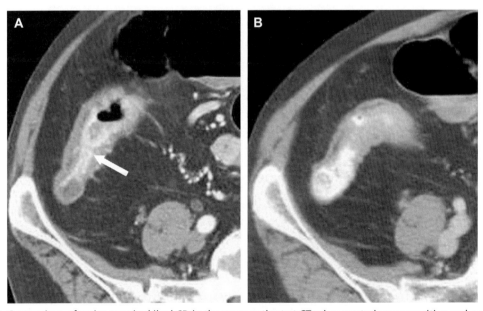

*Fig. 1.* Comparison of active terminal ileal CD in the same patient at CT using neutral versus positive oral contrast material. (*A*) Neutral oral contrast CTE. The increased mucosal enhancement (*arrow*) consistent with active CD can be identified easily using neutral intraluminal contrast. (*B*) Positive oral contrast CT. Note that the mucosal enhancement can no longer be identified because of the increased density of the positive oral contrast material.

rather than chronic disease [18,19]. Notably, CD has a predisposition to affect the mesenteric border of the small bowel. This asymmetric pattern of inflammation may create pseudosacculations or redundancy along the antimesenteric border [3].

Segmental mural hyperenhancement is another sign that correlates significantly with histologic [5,20] and clinical findings [18] of active CD. In fact, a recent study found that a semiautomated, quantitative analysis of mural attenuation using a threshold of 109 HU predicted active CD with a sensitivity similar to that of ileostomy [5]. The mural hyperenhancement seen with CD can have a variety of appearances. For example, the entire bowel wall can be thickened and enhancing, or there may be mural stratification demonstrating the layers of the bowel wall (Fig. 2).

Mural stratification in and of itself is also a reliable indicator for active CD [5,19,21], and at least one study found that it was more likely than a homogenously enhancing bowel wall to indicate histologically active CD [19]. Mural stratification patterns also can vary, having a bilaminar appearance with mucosal hyperenhancement and decreased intramural attenuation (Fig. 3) or a trilaminar appearance with mucosal and serosal hyperenhancement and decreased intramural enhancement (Fig. 4). The attenuation of the intramural portion of the bowel wall can vary depending on the pathologic process: the presence of intramural edema

(or water attenuation) indicates active inflammation, intramural soft tissue attenuation may represent an inflammatory infiltrate, and intramural fat usually indicates past or chronic inflammation (Fig. 5) [3].

Luminal narrowing is another common finding in CD and can be reversible or fixed. Small bowel luminal narrowing in CD is caused initially by mucosal edema and associated spasm. During this acute, noncicatrizing stage, the bowel wall is thickened and may display mural stratification (Fig. 6). Acute narrowing often is reversible with conservative measures and anti-inflammatory medications. With disease progression, the submucosa and smooth muscle layers become fibrotic, and strictures become fixed. This chronic fibrosis is demonstrated at CTE by homogenous enhancement of the bowel wall [22] or focal narrowing without significant wall thickening (Fig. 7). Fibrotic strictures must be treated with endoscopic dilation or surgical excision. Identifying the presence and type of stricture is important because the identification can determine therapy (medical versus surgical). In addition, capsule endoscopes are contraindicated in patients who have luminal narrowing less than 1 cm because of the risk of capsule retention that would require surgical removal. One study found that capsule retention occurred in 13% of patients who had known CD [23] and can cause intestinal perforation [24] and intestinal obstruction [25]. Thus, it has been suggested that before capsule endoscopy is

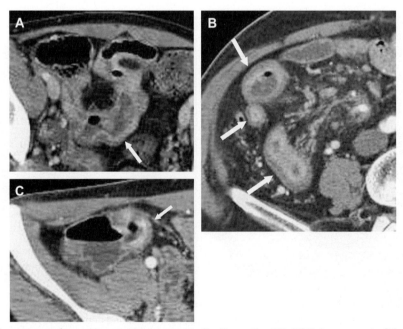

*Fig. 2.* Variable patterns of mural hyperenhancement indicating active CD. (*A*) Enhancement of the entire bowel wall (*arrow*). (*B*) Increased mucosal enhancement with submucosal edema (*arrows*), comb sign, and adenopathy. (*C*) Increased mucosal enhancement at the ileocolic anastomosis (*arrow*).

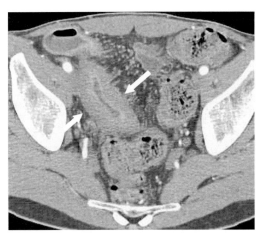

*Fig. 3.* Bilaminar stratification. Increased mucosal enhancement and intramural edema (*arrows*) hypervascularity consistent with active CD.

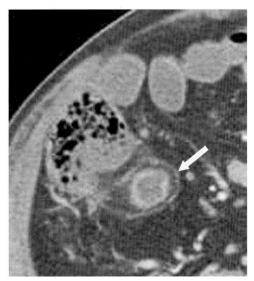

*Fig. 5.* Trilaminar stratification: chronic CD. Fatty intramural deposition (*arrow*) in a patient who has chronic CD.

used in the diagnosis of CD, a radiologic study be performed to exclude a stricture [26].

### Extraenteric findings

Extraenteric findings that are commonly seen at CD include the comb sign (Fig. 8), fibrofatty proliferation, fistulas (Fig. 9), and abscesses.

Engorged vasa recta that penetrate the bowel wall perpendicular to the bowel lumen create the comb sign. Although the comb sign does not seem to be a very sensitive finding in CD, it has been shown to be a very specific finding in active CD [5]. When present, engorged vasa recta correlate with clinically advanced, active, and extensive CD [12,27,28]. Specifically, it has been shown that patients with prominent vasculature had higher

C-reactive protein levels, were admitted to the hospital more frequently, and received a more intensive medication regimen more frequently than patients who had CD without prominent vasculature [27].

Fibrofatty proliferation can occur along the mesenteric border of bowel segments affected by CD and is considered to be surgically pathognomonic for the disease. Importantly, fibrofatty proliferation can be present in active and quiescent disease. Increased fat density, however, is a highly specific, although not particularly sensitive, finding for active CD [5]. Increased fat density is thought to indicate edema and inflammatory infiltration of the perienteric adipose tissue and has been correlated with histologic severity and serum C-reactive protein levels [12].

Extraenteric complications of transmural inflammation in CD include fistulas and abscesses. One population-based study found that for patients who have CD the cumulative risk of developing any fistula is 33% after 10 years and 50% after 20 years [29]. The most common type of fistula in CD is a perianal fistula, for which a cumulative risk after 20 years is estimated to be 26% [29]. Fistulas between parts of the gastrointestinal tract—enteroenteric, enterocolic, and colocolic—are common also and probably are underdiagnosed because they often are asymptomatic. Other types of fistulas that are seen more rarely in CD include enterocutaneous, rectovaginal, enterovaginal, and enterovesicular fistulas.

Fistulas generally are hyperenhancing tracts that arise from involved sections of bowel. Perianal fistulas, however, are an exception and typically are isoattenuating to the anorectum and often are

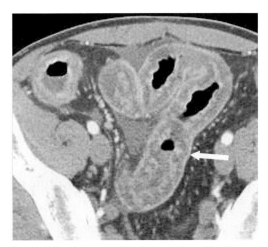

*Fig. 4.* Trilaminar stratification: active CD. Mucosal and serosal hyperemia with intramural edema (*arrow*) consistent with active CD.

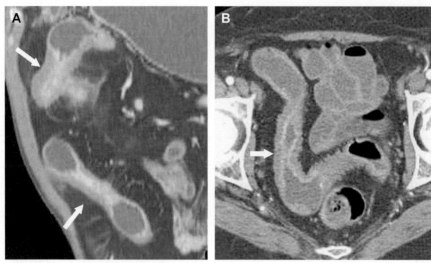

*Fig. 6. (A and B).* Reversible strictures. Narrowing of the bowel lumen caused by intramural edema (*arrows*) indicates these strictures are not yet fibrotic.

present in the absence of anal or rectal inflammation. No studies have compared the detection of fistulas by routine CT versus CTE. CTE may have an inherent advantage by using thinner slice collimation and generating higher-quality multiplanar reformatted images, but the use of positive oral contrast at routine CT may make fistula tracts more obvious. In the authors' practice, if a fistula is the main clinical question, they administer positive oral contrast but scan using the CTE protocol with multiplanar reformatted images.

Abscesses often are connected to inflamed bowel loops by a sinus tract and typically are found in the retroperitoneum or within the leaves of the mesentery [3]. Other extraenteric complications that are intrinsic to CD but seemingly unrelated to the inflammation of the bowel wall include sacroiliitis, renal stones, cholelithiasis, primary sclerosing cholangitis, and lymphoma.

### Differentiating underdistended normal bowel from diseased bowel

One potential pitfall in evaluation of the bowel wall for CD is confusing collapsed normal bowel for pathologic narrowing. The distinction can be particularly troublesome because poorly distended loops of bowel can appear both thickened and hyperenhancing. To problem solve, it is important to compare the attenuation of thickened small bowel loops with normal-appearing, distended bowel loops of the same bowel segment. Diseased bowel segments should appear hyperenhancing (because of bowel hyperemia) or hypoenhancing (because of bowel wall edema) compared with other loops in the same segment (Fig. 10). If the attenuation is similar, the finding probably represents underdistended normal bowel rather than disease (Fig. 11). It also is important to compare bowel loops in the same segment because the

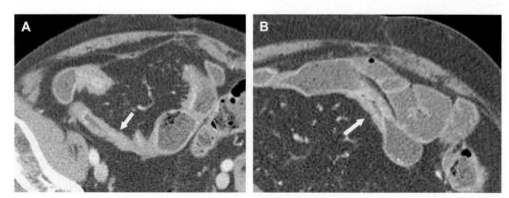

*Fig. 7.* Chronic, nonreversible strictures. (*A*) Narrowed stricture in the terminal ileum without significant wall thickening (*arrow*). (*B*) Second stricture in the ileum (*arrow*) with homogenous enhancing wall. Patient had undistensible and chronic strictures biopsied at endoscopy.

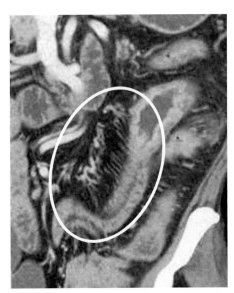

Fig. 8. Comb sign. Active CD with small bowel wall thickening and enhancement in the ileum with engorged vasa recta (comb sign) (*in circle*) extending to the bowel wall.

jejunum enhances to a greater extent than the ileum during scanning in the late arterial or enteric phase of enhancement (30–50 seconds after contrast material injection) (Fig. 12) [30]. In segments of bowel collapse, other signs of inflammation (ie, mural stratification, dilated vasculature, perienteric fat stranding, and increased density of the perienteric fat) must be relied upon. And, finally, rescanning through the relevant segment can be helpful.

### Performance of CT enterography in the evaluation of Crohn's disease

The difficulty in evaluating the performance of CTE for the detection of small bowel CD is the lack of a consistent criterion. Two methods have been devised to circumvent this problem. The first uses positive endoscopy and/or biopsy of the terminal ileum as the criterion for establishing the presence of CD [4,5]. This method is prone to false negatives, however, in patients in whom disease is proximal to the terminal ileum or in patients where the terminal ileum cannot be intubated. With this method, a positive CTE examination would be considered a false positive, regardless of how compelling radiologic assessment might be. It would be predictable that the specificity of CTE would suffer in this study design.

One of the studies that uses biopsy in the terminal ileum as a reference standard demonstrated an equivalent sensitivity for demonstration of active inflammation at the terminal ileum for CTE and ileoscopy (81% versus 81%), but, predictably, the specificity of CTE was significantly lower than that of ileoscopy (70% versus 97%) [5]. In the study by Wold and colleagues [4], a feasibility study with a relatively small number of patients, the sensitivity and specificity of multiple imaging tests were essentially equivalent: 78% and 83%, respectively for CTE, 75% and 100%, respectively, for CT enteroclysis, and 62% and 90%, respectively, for mall bowel follow through (SBFT). The CT examinations, however, were found to be more sensitive than SBFT in the detection of abscess, fistula, sacroiliitis, cholecystitis, and nephrolithiasis [4].

The second type of study design used to evaluate CD in the small bowel is one in which diagnostic yields are tabulated. In this study design, a positive finding by any modality is considered a true positive. The advantage of this method is that the performance of tests such as capsule endoscopy and CTE, which evaluate the small bowel outside the range of standard endoscopy, can be assessed. The disadvantage of this study design is that, because there is no reference standard, there is no way to detect a false positive, and calculation of the specificity is impossible. In addition, this method is at risk of overestimating disease prevalence and test sensitivity. For instance, many early studies of capsule endoscopy in patients who had CD showed that this test had a high diagnostic yield compared with barium examinations, suggesting that capsule endoscopy was a more sensitive test. Recently, however, findings suggestive of CD have been reported by capsule endoscopy in 10% to 21% of healthy controls [31,32]. In these same studies, positive findings were present in 55% to 71% of patients taking nonsteroidal anti-inflammatory drugs. These results suggest that studies of capsule endoscopy compared with other imaging techniques may have been overcalling rather than detecting true disease. This trade-off of high sensitivity for low specificity with capsule endoscopy has come under fire recently in the gastroenterology literature as being unacceptable, given the high penalty for a false positive in the diagnosis of CD [26].

Two studies compared CTE with other modalities using the diagnostic-yield study design. In the first, a prospective study by Hara and colleagues [33], CD was depicted by capsule endoscopy in 12 of 17 patients (71%), by ileoscopy in 11 of 17 patients (65%), by CTE in 9 of 17 patients (53%), and by SBFT in only 4 of 17 patients (24%). Despite the higher diagnostic yield for both capsule endoscopy and ileoscopy, this study highlighted some of the concerns with these modalities. In one of the 17 patients, SBFT failed to identify a small bowel stricture that resulted in a retained endoscopic capsule and required subsequent surgery for the removal of the capsule. Also, although experienced

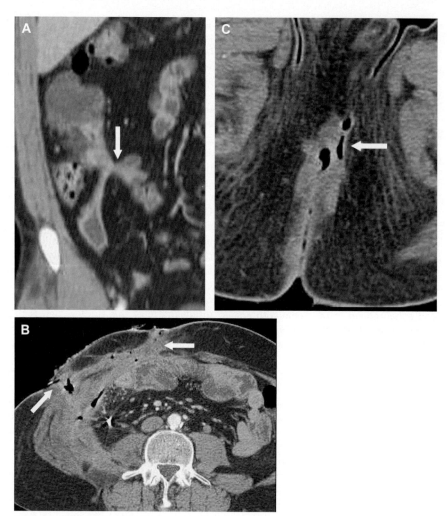

*Fig. 9.* Fistula types with CD. (*A*) Enteroenteric fistula (*arrow*) from the terminal ileum to a medial small bowel loop. (*B*) Multiple enterocutaneous fistulas (*arrows*). (*C*) Perianal fistula with an air-filled tract on the left (*arrow*).

gastroenterologists performed the ileoscopic examination, the terminal ileum was not intubated in 4 of 17 patients (24%), and capsule endoscopy did not visualize the terminal ileum in 2 of 17 patients (12%). The second study using diagnostic yield is a meta-analysis by Treister and colleagues [34] that compared capsule endoscopy with various modalities including CT. Notably, this study did not distinguish between CTE and CT enteroclysis. In this study the diagnostic yield for capsule endoscopy was 69%, and in the same group of patients the diagnostic yield of a CT examination was 30%.

## Obscure gastrointestinal bleeding

OGIB refers to the clinical presentation of recurrent or persistent gastrointestinal blood loss (visible fecal blood loss, positive fecal occult blood test, or iron

deficiency anemia) with no source of bleeding found at initial upper and lower endoscopy. Determining the origin of the bleeding source in OGIB is a challenging clinical problem. On average, in 27% of patients who have OGIB, the offending lesion causing the blood loss is located in the small bowel [35]. Small bowel vascular lesions are the most common cause, found in and 70% to 80% of OGIB cases [35]. The most common pathologic lesions in this group are angiodysplasias. Of unknown cause, these lesions are relatively common throughout the gastrointestinal tract and are found incidentally during colonoscopy in 2% of nonbleeding individuals over the age of 60 years. Small bowel tumors are the next most common small bowel lesion causing OGIB and account for 5% to 10% of all cases of small bowel bleeding. Although frank bleeding is a more common presentation for small bowel tumors,

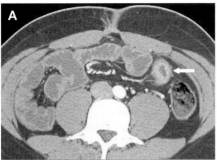
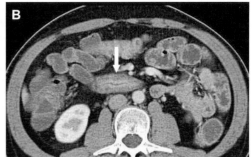

Fig. 10. Appearance of small bowel loops with active CD versus normal bowel loops. (A) Hyperenhancing (arrow) and thickened bowel loop compared with adjacent normal distended bowel. (B) Hypoenhancing bowel wall (arrow) caused by edema compared with normal enhancing adjacent bowel loops.

38% may present with a positive fecal occult blood test. Leiomyomas and gastrointestinal stromal tumors are the most common neoplasms causing OGIB, followed by adenomatous polyps, adenocarcinoma, lymphoma, and metastatic lesions. Other less common causes of bleeding include small bowel ulcers (eg, CD, use of nonsteroidal anti-inflammatory drugs, Meckel's diverticulum, vasculitis, small bowel diverticula, aortoenteric fistulas, and caliber-persistent arteries (Dieulafoy's lesion).

Capsule endoscopy has become the first-line diagnostic tool in evaluating patients who have OGIB. The sensitivity of capsule endoscopy for detection of small bowel lesions causing gastrointestinal bleeding ranges from 42% to 80% [36–41]. Capsule endoscopy is superior to both barium examination and extended endoscopy [42]. There are, however, certain disadvantages of capsule endoscopy: difficulty in localizing lesions, excessively long interpretation times (frequently > 75 minutes), a 1% to 2% incidence of intestinal obstruction caused by the device lodging behind a stricture, and occasional technical failure [43]. Currently, this technique is contraindicated in patients who have had previous major abdominal surgery, dysphagia, age younger than 18 years, or implanted cardiac pacemakers [44].

Multiphase CTE offers several advantages over capsule endoscopy. In addition to being less invasive and faster to perform, multiphase CTE allows visualization of the entire bowel wall, not just the mucosal surface. This ability is an important advantage over capsule endoscopy for detection of intramural bowel wall neoplasms that may not be visible on the mucosal surface. Furthermore, CTE allows examination of extraenteric structures and therefore provides a global examination of the abdomen.

## Imaging findings

The improved spatial resolution possible with 64-channel CT systems makes possible the detection

of minute abnormalities responsible for OGIB. Increased temporal resolution permits the use of multiphase scanning without sacrificing spatial resolution. Scanning during multiple phases increases the likelihood of detection of vascular lesions that may be visible only transiently. In addition, the depiction of the evolving nature of the abnormalities on sequential phases may provide clues to the nature of the abnormality. Furthermore, visualization of an abnormality during multiple phases increases diagnostic confidence.

The detection of abnormalities causing OGIB requires careful examination of each scanning phase depicted in multiple planes. Coping with this massive volume of image data requires a workstation capable of displaying multiple phases and imaging planes simultaneously.

The imaging findings in OGIB depend on the nature of the lesion responsible for the bleeding. Benign vascular abnormalities, including angiodysplasias, are responsible for most cases of OGIB. The multiphase CTE appearance of these lesions is similar to the angiographic appearance reported by

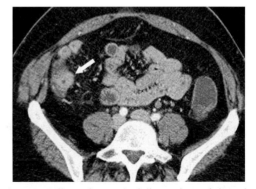

Fig. 11. Collapsed, terminal ileum (arrow) has the same attenuation as adjacent bowel loops indicating the apparent thickening is caused by underdistention rather than CD. Patient had a negative ileoscopy.

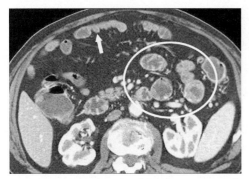

*Fig. 12.* Normal jejunum (*circle*) enhances more than distal small bowel (*arrow*) during the arterial phase. This increased enhancement should not be confused with CD. Notice the absence of bowel wall edema and hypervascularity.

Boley and colleagues [45]. Common findings include the presence of a vascular tuft visible during the arterial phase and an early draining mesenteric vein (Fig. 13). The vascular tuft may be very small, in the range of 2 to 10 mm [46]. It may appear as a focal irregular area of enhancement or an ectatic vessel in the bowel wall. The detection of an early draining vein should encourage a more careful search for a vascular nidus in the adjacent bowel wall.

Active bleeding appears as the progressive accumulation of contrast in the dependent portion of the bowel lumen (Fig. 14). The evolving appearance of active bleeding can be appreciated only during multiphasic scanning. Bleeding from angiodysplastic lesions is most likely intermittent; therefore active bleeding is less commonly seen in stable patients.

An unusual cause of OGIB is a venous angioma of the small bowel (Fig. 15). The authors have seen two such cases in patients who have OGIB.

In both cases, the gradual accumulation of contrast was noted within ectatic venous channels within the bowel wall, a pattern not dissimilar to theenhancement pattern commonly seen in hepatic cavernous hemangiomas.

The CT appearance of small bowel tumors has been described adequately in the literature [47]. Gastrointestinal stromal tumors are associated most commonly with OGIB and appear as brightly enhancing bowel wall masses visible during the arterial and enteric phases, tending to become less intense during delayed phases. When large, they tend to have large feeding arteries and draining veins. These tumors frequently do not disturb the mucosal surface and therefore may not be detected by wireless capsule endoscopy.

A variety of other abnormalities are less common causes of OGIB. Among these lesions, CD is the most common and has been discussed previously.

### Performance of CT enterography in the evaluation of obscure gastrointestinal bleeding

In a recent study, 22 stable outpatients who had OGIB (hematochezia, melena, or Hemoccult-positive stools) underwent a timed, multiphase CTE examination [11]. Multiphase CTE was positive for active bleeding or focal bowel abnormality thought to be a bleeding source in 10 of 22 of cases (45%). Nine of 10 positive multiphase CTE patients underwent capsule endoscopy. Multiphase CTE correctly identified a jejunal stromal tumor, a cecal arteriovenous malformation (subsequently successfully embolized), and a vascular jejunal wall mass (confirmed on a repeat capsule endoscopy study 5 months later), all of which were missed by capsule endoscopy.

Multiphase CTE was negative in 12 of 22 patients. Of these 12, only 4 underwent capsule endoscopy,

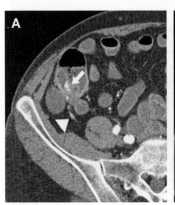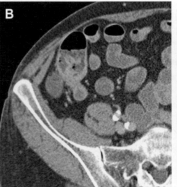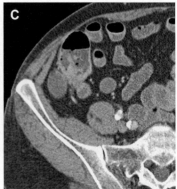

*Fig. 13.* Cecal angiodysplasia. (*A*) Vascular tuft (*arrow*) and early draining mesenteric vein (*arrowhead*) during arterial phase. No abnormalities are visible on the (*B*) enteric and (*C*) delayed phases.

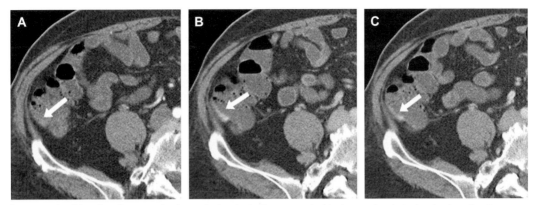

*Fig. 14.* Active bleeding from a colonic angiodysplasia demonstrated by increasing intraluminal contrast accumulation (*arrows*) during (*A*) arterial, (*B*) enteric, and (*C*) delayed phases.

and a small bowel lesion (jejunal lymphangioma) was localized by capsule endoscopy in only 1 patient. A second patient had small bowel blood, determined to originate in a hiatal hernia at subsequent endoscopy, resulting from Cameron's ulcers. Although the results are preliminary, the evidence suggests that multiphase CTE may play a complementary role to conventional and capsule endoscopy in evaluating OGIB.

## Pitfalls of CT enterography

Inadequate bowel distention at CTE can be caused by several factors including patient noncompliance with ingesting the oral contrast, delays in CT access (ie, scanner running late), history of small bowel resection, delayed gastric emptying, gastric outlet or small bowel obstruction, or small bowel motility disorders. In patients who have a history of small bowel resection, it can be helpful to image earlier

after oral contrast administration (30 minutes) rather than at 45 minutes. In addition, it is important to ensure that the patient can receive intravenous contrast, because this is a critical part of assessing for abnormal inflammation or masses. If the patient cannot receive intravenous contrast, positive oral contrast should be given for better evaluation of the small bowel. As discussed previously, in some cases, identification of fistulas may be improved with positive rather than neutral oral contrast. Finally, some patients experience nausea or diarrhea because of the barium solution.

## Summary

CT enterography is a noninvasive imaging test using neutral intraluminal contrast and intravenous contrast to evaluate the small bowel.

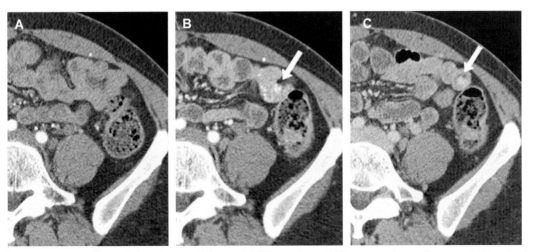

*Fig. 15.* Venous angioma of the jejunum. (*A*) Arterial, (*B*) enteric, and (*C*) venous phases show gradual contrast accumulation within angioma (*arrows* in panels *B* and *C*).

Multiphasic imaging (arterial, enteric, delayed) is used for the evaluation of OGIB, and single-phase enteric imaging is used for all other indications, including CD.

CTE imaging findings of CD include bowel wall thickening, mucosal hyperenhancement, and mural stratification.

CTE imaging findings of angiodysplasias include a vascular tuft visible during the arterial phase and an early draining mesenteric vein.

Early studies indicate that CTE is superior to barium exams in the evaluation of CD and is complementary to capsule endoscopy in the evaluation of OGIB.

## References

[1] Fishman EK, Wolf EJ, Jones B, et al. CT evaluation of Crohn's disease: effect on patient management. AJR Am J Roentgenol 1987;148:537–40.

[2] Raptopoulos V, Schwartz RK, McNicholas MM, et al. Multiplanar helical CT enterography in patients with Crohn's disease. AJR Am J Roentgenol 1997;169:1545–50.

[3] Paulsen SR, Huprich JE, Fletcher JG, et al. CT enterography as a diagnostic tool in evaluating small bowel disorders: review of clinical experience with over 700 cases. Radiographics 2006; 26:641–57 [discussion: 657–62].

[4] Wold PB, Fletcher JG, Johnson CD, et al. Assessment of small bowel Crohn disease: noninvasive peroral CT enterography compared with other imaging methods and endoscopy–feasibility study. Radiology 2003;229:275–81.

[5] Bodily KD, Fletcher JG, Solem CA, et al. Crohn disease: mural attenuation and thickness at contrast-enhanced CT enterography—correlation with endoscopic and histologic findings of inflammation. Radiology 2006;238:505–16.

[6] Megibow AJ, Babb JS, Hecht EM, et al. Evaluation of bowel distention and bowel wall appearance by using neutral oral contrast agent for multidetector row CT. Radiology 2006;238:87–95.

[7] Arslan H, Etlik O, Kayan M, et al. Peroral CT enterography with lactulose solution: preliminary observations. AJR Am J Roentgenol 2005;185: 1173–9.

[8] Oliva MR, Erturk S, Ichikawa T, et al. Abdominal MDCT with neutral oral contrast media (VoLumen): comparison with positive oral contrast media and water [abstract No. SSJ06-03]. Presented at the annual meeting of the Radiological Society of North America. Chicago, November 29, 2005.

[9] Al-Hawary M, Platt J, Francis I. Comparison of adequacy of oral contrast bowel preparation with two different low attenuation agents for CT enterography in patients with known or suspected inflammatory bowel disease [abstract No. SSJ06-02]. Presented at the annual meeting

of the Radiological Society of North America. Chicago, November 29, 2005.

[10] Young BM, Fletcher JG, Paulsen SR. Comparison of oral contrast agents for cross-sectional enterography: timing, small bowel distention, and side effects. Presented at the annual meeting of the Society of Gastrointestinal Radiologists. San Antonio (TX), February 28, 2005.

[11] Huprich JE. Obscure GI bleeding: 64 channel, multi-phase, multiplanar CT enterography has a role [abstract No. SSM09-06]. Presented at the annual meeting of the Radiological Society of North America. Chicago, November 30, 2005.

[12] Colombel JF, Solem CA, Sandborn WJ, et al. Quantitative measurement and visual assessment of ileal Crohn's disease activity by CT enterography: correlation with endoscopic severity and C-reactive protein. Gut 2006;55(11): 1561–7.

[13] Horton KM, Eng J, Fishman EK. Normal enhancement of the small bowel: evaluation with spiral CT. J Comput Assist Tomogr 2000;24:67–71.

[14] Angelelli G, Macarini L. CT of the bowel: use of water to enhance depiction. Radiology 1988; 169:848–9.

[15] Rollandi GA, Curone PF, Biscaldi E, et al. Spiral CT of the abdomen after distention of small bowel loops with transparent enema in patients with Crohn's disease. Abdom Imaging 1999;24: 544–9.

[16] Sands BE. Crohn's disease. In: Feldman M, Friedman L, Sleisenger M, editors. Sleisenger and Fordtran's gastrointestinal and liver disease. Philidelphia: Saunders; 2002. p. 2005–38.

[17] Maccioni F, Bruni A, Viscido A, et al. MR imaging in patients with Crohn disease: value of T2- versus T1-weighted gadolinium-enhanced MR sequences with use of an oral superparamagnetic contrast agent. Radiology 2006;238: 517–30.

[18] Del Campo L, Arribas I, Valbuena M, et al. Spiral CT findings in active and remission phases in patients with Crohn disease. J Comput Assist Tomogr 2001;25:792–7.

[19] Choi D, Jin Lee S, Ah Cho Y, et al. Bowel wall thickening in patients with Crohn's disease: CT patterns and correlation with inflammatory activity. Clin Radiol 2003;58:68–74.

[20] Booya F, Fletcher JG, Johnson CD, et al. CT enterography: detection of active Crohn's disease during optimal bowel wall enhancement [abstract]. In: Program of the Radiological Society of North America scientific assembly and annual meeting. Chicago: Radiological Society of North America; 2004. p. 611.

[21] Mako EK, Mester AR, Tarjan Z, et al. Enteroclysis and spiral CT examination in diagnosis and evaluation of small bowel Crohn's disease. Eur J Radiol 2000;35:168–75.

[22] Gore RM, Balthazar EJ, Ghahremani GG, et al. CT features of ulcerative colitis and Crohn's disease. AJR Am J Roentgenol 1996;167:3–15.

[23] Cheifetz AS, Kornbluth AA, Legnani P, et al. The risk of retention of the capsule endoscope in patients with known or suspected Crohn's disease. Am J Gastroenterol 2006;101(10):2218–22.

[24] Gonzalez Carro P, Picazo Yuste J, Fernandez Diez S, et al. Intestinal perforation due to retained wireless capsule endoscope. Endoscopy 2005;37:684.

[25] Gay G, Delvaux M, Laurent V, et al. Temporary intestinal occlusion induced by a "patency capsule" in a patient with Crohn's disease. Endoscopy 2005;37:174–7.

[26] Lashner BA. Sensitivity-specificity trade-off for capsule endoscopy in IBD: is it worth it? Am J Gastroenterol 2006;101:965–6.

[27] Lee SS, Ha HK, Yang SK, et al. CT of prominent pericolic or perienteric vasculature in patients with Crohn's disease: correlation with clinical disease activity and findings on barium studies. AJR Am J Roentgenol 2002;179:1029–36.

[28] Meyers MA, McGuire PV. Spiral CT demonstration of hypervascularity in Crohn disease: "vascular jejunization of the ileum" or the "comb sign". Abdom Imaging 1995;20:327–32.

[29] Schwartz DA, Loftus EV Jr, Tremaine WJ, et al. The natural history of fistulizing Crohn's disease in Olmsted County, Minnesota. Gastroenterology 2002;122:875–80.

[30] Booya F, Fletcher JG, Johnson CD, et al. Conspicuity of small bowel inflammation at CT enterography: "enteric" vs. "hepatic" phase imaging. [abstract]. In: Program of the Radiological Society of North America scientific assembly and annual meeting. Chicago: Radiological Society of North America; 2004. p. 611.

[31] Graham DY, Opekun AR, Willingham FF, et al. Visible small-intestinal mucosal injury in chronic NSAID users. Clin Gastroenterol Hepatol 2005; 3:55–9.

[32] Goldstein JL, Eisen GM, Lewis B, et al. Video capsule endoscopy to prospectively assess small bowel injury with celecoxib, naproxen plus omeprazole, and placebo. Clin Gastroenterol Hepatol 2005;3:133–41.

[33] Hara AK, Leighton JA, Heigh RI, et al. Crohn disease of the small bowel: preliminary comparison among CT enterography, capsule endoscopy, small-bowel follow-through, and ileoscopy. Radiology 2006;238:128–34.

[34] Triester SL, Leighton JA, Leontiadis GI, et al. A meta-analysis of the yield of capsule endoscopy compared to other diagnostic modalities in patients with non-stricturing small bowel Crohn's disease. Am J Gastroenterol 2006;101:954–64.

[35] Lahoti S, Fukami N. The small bowel as a source of gastrointestinal blood loss. Curr Gastroenterol Rep 1999;1:424–30.

[36] Adler DG, Knipschield M, Gostout C. A prospective comparison of capsule endoscopy and push enteroscopy in patients with GI bleeding of obscure origin. Gastrointest Endosc 2004;59: 492–8.

[37] Ell C, Remke S, May A, et al. The first prospective controlled trial comparing wireless capsule endoscopy with push enteroscopy in chronic gastrointestinal bleeding. Endoscopy 2002;34: 685–9.

[38] Mata A, Bordas JM, Feu F, et al. Wireless capsule endoscopy in patients with obscure gastrointestinal bleeding: a comparative study with push enteroscopy. Aliment Pharmacol Ther 2004;20: 189–94.

[39] Pennazio M, Santucci R, Rondonotti E, et al. Outcome of patients with obscure gastrointestinal bleeding after capsule endoscopy: report of 100 consecutive cases [see comment]. Gastroenterology 2004;126:643–53.

[40] Magnano A, Privitera A, Calogero G, et al. The role of capsule endoscopy in the work-up of obscure gastrointestinal bleeding. Eur J Gastroenterol Hepatol 2004;16:403–6.

[41] Scapa E, Jacob H, Lewkowicz S, et al. Initial experience of wireless-capsule endoscopy for evaluating occult gastrointestinal bleeding and suspected small bowel pathology. Am J Gastroenterol 2002; 97:2776–9.

[42] Ge ZZ, Hu YB, Xiao SD. Capsule endoscopy and push enteroscopy in the diagnosis of obscure gastrointestinal bleeding. Chin Med J 1045; 117:1045–49.

[43] Arnott ID, Lo SK. The clinical utility of wireless capsule endoscopy. Dig Dis Sci 2004;49:893–901.

[44] Fireman Z, Kopelman Y. The role of video capsule endoscopy in the evaluation of iron deficiency anaemia. Dig Liver Dis 2004;36:97–102.

[45] Boley S, Sprayregen S, Sammartano R, et al. The pathophysiologic basis for the angiographic signs of vascular ectasias of the colon. Radiology 1977;125:615–21.

[46] Lewis BS. Vascular diseases of the small intestine. In: DiMarino A, Benjamin S, editors. Gastrointestinal disease: an endoscopic approach. Malden (MA): Blackwell Science; 1997. p. 541–50.

[47] Horton KM, Juluru K, Montogomery E, et al. Computed tomography imaging of gastrointestinal stromal tumors with pathology correlation. J Comput Assist Tomogr 2004;28:811–7.

RADIOLOGIC
CLINICS
OF NORTH AMERICA

ELSEVIER
SAUNDERS

Radiol Clin N Am 45 (2007) 317–331

# MR Imaging of the Small Bowel

Jeff Fidler, MD

- Advantages
- Limitations
- Technical issues
  - *Enteroclysis versus enterography*
  - *Enteric contrast agents*
  - *Pulse sequences*
- Indications
  - *Assessment of Crohn's disease*
  - *Small bowel obstruction*
  - *Small bowel neoplasms*
- Summary
- References

The small bowel is the last great frontier in gastrointestinal luminal evaluation. Endoscopic techniques can access the stomach and colon easily, and these techniques now are used widely for diagnosis and treatment of abnormalities in these organs. The use of endoscopy for evaluation of the small bowel is limited, however, because of its location and length. There has been tremendous interest in developing new methods that will allow improved accuracy for the detection of small bowel pathology. Historically, barium techniques, small bowel series, and fluoroscopic enteroclysis have been the only techniques available to examine the small bowel in its entirety. The results of these barium studies for certain abnormalities have been disappointing. Newer techniques, such as wireless capsule endoscopy, push endoscopy, and double-balloon enteroscopy, have been developed to fill this imaging void. Advances in computer technology have allowed cross-sectional imaging techniques to play a larger role in the imaging of small bowel disorders, and in the author's practice the volume of cross-sectional enterography examinations currently outnumber barium examinations of the small bowel. Improvements in CT and MR imaging technology have led to improved spatial and temporal resolution that now allows exquisite high-resolution imaging using enterography and enteroclysis techniques. In the next few years

ongoing studies comparing these new and evolving techniques for imaging the small bowel will be needed to determine appropriate work-up algorithms using state-of-the-art equipment.

Cross-sectional imaging techniques such as CT and MR imaging have advantages over traditional barium fluoroscopic techniques in their ability to visualize superimposed bowel loops better and to improve visualization of extraluminal findings and complications. This article discusses MR imaging of the small bowel with enterography and enteroclysis techniques. It reviews the advantages, limitations, technique, and indications and reviews the results that have been obtained in evaluating different disease processes.

## Advantages

MR imaging has many unique properties that make it well suited for imaging the gastrointestinal tract. These properties include the lack of ionizing radiation, the improved tissue contrast that can be obtained by using a variety of pulse sequences and parameters, the ability to perform real-time and functional imaging, and the safety profile of gadolinium contrast agents.

CT can obtain exquisite high-resolution images of the small bowel but at a cost of radiation exposure to the patient. There is controversy about the

The author has received research support from E-Z-EM, Inc.
Department of Radiology, Mayo Clinic, 200 First Street SW, Rochester, MN 55905, USA
*E-mail address:* fidler.jeff@mayo.edu

doi:10.1016/j.rcl.2007.03.012

significance of this amount of radiation exposure. Several disease processes that affect the small bowel, such as Crohn's disease and the polyposis syndromes, occur in younger patients who may require frequent imaging for surveillance. Therefore, the cumulative amount of lifetime radiation exposure for these patients may not be trivial. Thus, imaging surveillance that can be performed without ionizing radiation would be very beneficial to these patients.

Because of the intrinsic properties of MR imaging, soft tissue contrast is better than with CT. This difference may be important for detecting subtle areas of pathology and may improve characterization of certain abnormalities. One area in which improved soft-tissue contrast has been shown to be helpful is in the evaluation of perianal fistulas in the setting of Crohn's disease. MR imaging has been shown to correlate well in detecting and staging these fistulas and in the author's practice is the preferred technique to detect, stage, and follow perianal fistulizing disease [1–4]. Thus, the examination for perianal fistulas could be combined with examination of the small bowel and, potentially, colon to assess the entire gastrointestinal tract and provide a comprehensive examination with one imaging modality.

MR imaging also offers the ability to provide a functional or real-time examination of the bowel [5]; because of ionizing radiation exposure at CT, imaging can be obtained at only a few points in time. This limitation may cause difficulty in determining if areas of bowel narrowing are secondary to contractions or to fixed strictures. Bowel peristalsis and distensibility can be evaluated easily with MR imaging by using multiphase imaging techniques or MR fluoroscopy without the concern for radiation exposure. These techniques can be helpful in evaluating the progress of bowel filling with contrast agents during enteroclysis to allow optimal timing of imaging. The real-time imaging also can help determine the distensibility of narrowed areas and improve differentiation of contractions from strictures (Fig. 1).

The gadolinium contrast agents used in MR imaging have an excellent safety profile and can be administered in patients who have iodine contrast allergies or renal insufficiency, overcoming some of the limitations of CT.

## Limitations

Although several advantages make MR imaging ideally suited to image the small bowel, several limitations have prevented more widespread clinical implementation.

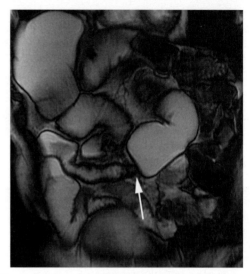

*Fig. 1.* Small bowel obstruction. Coronal image from a multiphase 2D TrueFISP sequence using enterography technique shows a transition point (*arrow*) in this patient with symptoms of intermittent low-grade small bowel obstruction. The multiphase technique allows assessment of the distensibility of areas of narrowing (see video. Access mmc1.video in online version of article at http://www.radiologic.theclinics.com.)

One of the main limitations is the inferior spatial and temporal resolution in comparison with CT. Using multidetector CT scanners, 2- to 3-mm images can be obtained quickly throughout the abdomen in a single breath and allow exquisite demonstration of the abdominal contents. With this improved spatial resolution, multiplanar reformatted images can be generated in various planes. In comparison, the slice thickness for MR imaging is usually 4 to 6 mm, and some of the sequences require a few separate breath-holds. Parallel imaging techniques have been developed and can be used with some sequences to reduce scan times to a single breath-hold with a trade-off in the signal-to-noise ratio [6]. Improved temporal resolution reduces artifacts from bowel peristalsis that can degrade image quality on MR imaging. The improved spatial and temporal resolution of CT over MR imaging does not necessarily translate into improved sensitivity and specificity, however. More research is needed comparing state-of-the-art MR imaging with CT techniques in the various disorders of the small bowel to determine what resolution is required to obtain adequate sensitivity and specificities. Thus, there is a balance when comparing CT and MR imaging for imaging the small bowel. One must determine if the lack of ionizing radiation, functional information, and soft tissue contrast that can be obtained with MR imaging outweigh the inferior spatial and temporal resolution.

Another limitation in the United States is the medical community's perception about exposure to ionizing radiation. Many of the studies that have been published assessing MR imaging have been performed in European countries where there is more emphasis on using imaging techniques without ionizing radiation. Until there is a greater emphasis on avoiding exposure to ionizing radiation in this country, the shift to non-ionizing radiating techniques probably will be delayed.

Scanner access also may limit the implementation of MR imaging. In many practices there are limited numbers of MR scanners and examination slots. Currently, the majority of MR imaging examinations performed in most practices consist of neurologic and musculoskeletal indications. Abdominal applications are increasing but mainly for imaging the solid organs of the abdomen. Luminal imaging must compete for these examination times. In many practices the scheduling access to cross-sectional techniques is easier for CT because of the relatively greater number of CT scanners. Also the overall examination time is faster with CT than with MR imaging, and thus more examinations can be performed during the same period with CT than with MR imaging.

The slow implementation of MR imaging of the small bowel in clinical practice may be influenced by the radiologists who are performing the examination. In many practices the gastrointestinal radiologists are the radiologists who are actively involved with the gastroenterologists in the assessment of patients suspected of having small bowel disorders and in recommending appropriate imaging algorithms. Most gastrointestinal radiologists are involved in barium fluoroscopy and CT; however, in many practices not all of these radiologists may be involved in the MR imaging practice. In addition, in many practices the individuals who are performing MR imaging may be too busy developing other parts of the MR imaging practice and thus may not be interested or able to develop gastrointestinal luminal–specific protocols. It is imperative that these two groups of individuals work together closely so that appropriate education on indications, advantages, and limitations of MR imaging are realized fully by the radiologists and clinicians.

The costs associated with an MR imaging examination also may hinder widespread acceptance of the technique. Cross-sectional imaging techniques are significantly more expensive than traditional barium examinations. Further studies assessing the cost effectiveness of these more expensive techniques are needed.

## Technical issues

### Enteroclysis versus enterography

Most of the studies published to date on MR imaging of the small bowel have been performed with enteroclysis techniques. Enteroclysis requires intubation of the duodenum or proximal small bowel with the administration of enteric contrast agents. The intubation usually is performed under fluoroscopy. The small bowel then can be filled while the patient is in the scanner, using manual injection or hand-held infusion pumps. Automated pumps can be adapted and used at a distance from the bore of the magnet. The progress of small bowel filling can be monitored using MR fluoroscopy or by repeating thick-slab half-Fourier acquisition single-shot turbo echo-spin (HASTE) images. Alternatively, the small bowel can be filled outside the scanner; however continuous infusion provides the best small bowel distension.

Enterography techniques require the ingestion of a large amount of fluid (1.5–2 L) that fills the stomach and the small bowel in continuity. Enterography obviates the need for nasoenteric intubation and thus has better patient acceptance than enteroclysis. Although enteroclysis techniques theoretically provide better small bowel distention, there is a paucity of data available comparing the sensitivity of enteroclysis and enterography in various small bowel disorders.

Two studies have been published comparing enteroclysis and enterography in patients who have Crohn's disease. In a study of 21 patients, MR enterography and MR enteroclysis were performed in the same patients after conventional enteroclysis. In this study all pathologic findings seen on conventional enteroclysis were seen on MR enterography and MR enteroclysis. MR imaging detected additional information in 6 of 21 patients [7]. In another study of 23 patients suspected of having Crohn's disease, patients were examined using either enterography or enteroclysis techniques by CT. This study showed similar degrees of distention in these two groups, and there was similar accuracy for detecting active Crohn's disease [8]. Thus it may be possible to obtain adequate results with enterographic techniques alone, obviating the need for nasoenteric intubation. Further studies are needed to determine if enterography compares favorably with enteroclysis. In the author's practice, he and his colleagues have chosen to perform enterography as the routine technique for both CT and MR imaging, reserving enteroclysis for select indications such as low-grade small bowel obstruction when needed.

## Enteric contrast agents

Enteric contrast agents can be classified according to their appearance on the T1- and T2-weighted pulse sequences. Negative contract agents produce low signal intensity on T1- and T2-weighted images. Positive contrast agents produce high signal intensity on T1- and T2-weighted images. Biphasic contrast agents are low signal intensity on one sequence and high signal intensity on the opposite sequence. The majority of biphasic contrast agents have low signal intensity on the T1-weighted image and high signal intensity on the T2-weighted image.

### Negative contrast agents

Negative contrast agents consist of the superparamagnetic particles such as perfluorooctyl bromide, ferumoxide oral suspension, and oral magnetic particles [9–14]. These agents have a small incidence of side effects that can be seen in 5% to 15% of cases and are related mainly to the gastrointestinal tract: the less-than-optimal palatability of the agent, nausea, vomiting, and rectal leakage. Gas potentially can be used as a negative contrast agent, but it may be difficult to fill the small bowel in its entirety. High weight per volume barium also can lower the signal intensity of the lumen, but the signal loss is not as great as with the superparamagnetic particles.

Limitations of the negative contrast agents include the side effects mentioned previously, imaging artifacts that can occur (especially with the use of lower field strength magnets), and the price of the agent. If these agents are not distributed homogenously throughout the bowel, they can produce paradoxical high signal intensity.

Bowel wall thickening can be demonstrated exquisitely on T1-weighted images using these agents. Also, because these agents have low signal intensity on T1-weighted images, bowel wall enhancement is well demonstrated. The high signal intensity of inflammation in the bowel wall and surrounding fat may be more conspicuous on T2-weighted images using negative contrast agents, because there is greater contrast between the inflammation and the low signal intensity lumen. These agents may improve the conspicuity of inner-loop abscess. The negative contrast agent decreases the signal intensity in the bowel lumen but not the high signal intensity abscess on T2-weighted images (Fig. 2).

### Positive contrast agents

Positive contrast agents consist of the paramagnetic substances such as the gadolinium chelates, manganese ions, and ferrous ions [9,11]. Many natural substances have been investigated including milk, vegetable oil, ice cream, green tea, and blueberry juice [15]. As with the negative contrast agents,

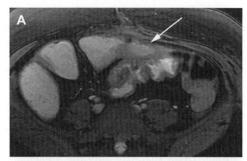

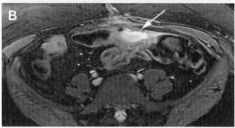

*Fig. 2.* Inner-loop abscess in Crohn's disease. Axial T2-weighted 2D TrueFISP images with fat suppression from MR enterography using (*A*) biphasic enteric contrast and (*B*) negative enteric contrast show an inner-loop abscess (*arrows*) in a patient who has Crohn's disease. Note the improved conspicuity with the negative enteric contrast in panel B.

side effects are seen in a small percentage of patients. Limitations of the natural substances relate to the ability to store these agents and administer them in a busy clinical practice.

Positive contrast agents also demonstrate wall thickening well on T1-weighted images. A limitation related to these contrast agents is that the high signal intensity produced in the lumen may mask the detection of enhancement of the bowel wall or intraluminal masses after administration of intravenous contrast.

Positive contrast agents also can increase the conspicuity of inner-loop abscesses. With positive contrast agents, the bowel lumen will have high signal intensity on T1-weighted images, and inner-loop abscesses maintain their low signal intensity fluid with rim enhancement.

In one study investigators compared both positive and negative enteric contrast agents in combination with enteroclysis. Patients were assigned randomly to receive either a positive or negative enteric contrast agent. Twenty-seven patients had Crohn's disease, and two had small bowel tumors. The detection of fistulas was not influenced by the choice of the enteric contrast agent. The diagnosis of abscesses and the contrast between the wall and lumen was influenced by the choice of oral contrast agent. If positive oral contrast medium was used, abscesses were detected best on T1-weighted postcontrast sequences. If negative oral contrast was used, T2-weighted sequences were the most useful. On T2-weighted images, the contrast between the wall and the positive oral contrast agents was only moderately good in six cases because of the edema and inflamed intestinal wall. With negative oral contrast media, the contrast between the wall and lumen was found to be less satisfactory. The inflamed bowel segment was detected in all cases. The use of intravenous contrast medium significantly improved contrast from the inflamed bowel wall [9].

### Biphasic contrast agents

Many agents in the biphasic category have been assessed. Each of these agents has unique limitations. Water has been used in high volumes over a short ingestion period [16]. Water, however, is absorbed rapidly from the distal small bowel, and adequate distention may not be obtained. Osmotic agents such as mannitol have been evaluated [17,18]. Potential limitations with this agent are the formation of gas and the osmotic effects. Non-osmotic agents such as locust bean gum and methylcellulose have been evaluated [18,19]. These agents, however, are not widely available. Methylcellulose was manufactured for administration during enteroclysis techniques; thus the taste and consistency are not optimal. Polyethylene glycol, a cathartic widely used for colonoscopy preparation, is a non-osmotic agent [20–23] that provides excellent distension but also leads to rapid diarrhea and a strong urge for evacuation that can interfere with the completion of the examination. A rectal tube can be inserted before the examination to prevent accidental evacuation, allow decompression of the rectum, and subsequently decrease the urge to evacuate. Barium products at lower weight per volume also can act as biphasic agents. Manganese agents were developed commercially but are no longer available. Water-soluble iodinated contrast agents such as a diatrizoate meglumine and diatrizoate sodium solution also have been evaluated [24,25]. Limitations relate to the taste of this agent and the associated diarrhea that can occur. This agent does not produce as high signal intensity as simple fluid on the T2-weighted images. Concentrated gadolinium chelates mixed with barium have been assessed. These agents provide the opposite signal intensity of the biphasic agents mentioned previously; they have high signal intensity on T1-weighted images and low signal on T2-weighted images [26].

Many of the negative and positive contrast agents that were developed commercially are no longer available. The author and colleagues have implemented neutral contrast agents into their CT enterography practice. These agents allow improved conspicuity of enhancement in the bowel wall and lumen, which is important for detecting active inflammation, enhancing masses, and sites of bleeding. These agents are easy to administer and are widely available. The neutral contrast agents that are used for CT provide biphasic characteristics on MR imaging, and the low signal intensity on the T1-weighted images allows excellent demonstration of enhancement. The author and colleagues have evaluated and implemented the enteric contrast agents used for CT in their MR imaging practice, encouraging more standardized practice in the administration of an enteric contrast agent.

The author and colleagues have evaluated four main agents in their CT and MR imaging practice: water, methylcellulose, polyethylene glycol, and a low Hounsfield-value barium that is available commercially for CT. As indicated previously, water is absorbed rapidly from the distal bowel and does not provide adequate distention. Methylcellulose is no longer available. Polyethylene glycol can be administered and provides excellent distension, but with this agent the urge to evacuate can be fairly great, and it may be difficult to complete an entire MR imaging examination. In the author's experience the low Hounsfield-value barium provides good distention and is well tolerated by patients. The author and colleagues have incorporated this agent into their CT and MR imaging practice because of the quality of distension, ease in administration, and patient tolerance. Continued research is needed to optimize bowel distension further.

### Pulse sequences

Several different pulse sequences are available for imaging the small bowel. The main diagnostic sequences can be divided into the T2-weighted sequences that consist of the single-shot HASTE techniques (single-shot fast spin echo [SSFSE], HASTE, single-shot turbo spin echo) and the balanced gradient echo (Fast Imaging Employing Steady-State Acquisition, True Fast Imaging with Steady-state Precession [FISP], balanced fast field echo) sequences. Contrast enhanced T1-weighted gradient echo sequences with fat suppression also are routinely performed to look for areas of increased enhancement. These can be performed as either two-dimensional (2D) (fast spoiled grass, Turbo fast low angle shot, turbo field echo) or three-dimensional (3D) (Fast Acquisition with Multiphase Efgre 3D, Volumetric Interpolated Breath-hold Examination, T1 High Resolution Isotropic Volume Examination) sequences. Fast T1-weighted gradient echo sequences without fat suppression or T1-weighted fast spin echo sequences also can be performed before intravenous contrast injection to aid in detecting and characterizing abnormalities. Fat-suppression techniques can be helpful in T2-weighted images by showing increased conspicuity of high signal intensity in the bowel wall and mesenteric fat in areas of active inflammation [27]. Parallel imaging has allowed a significant decrease in scan times. Parallel imaging takes advantage of the spatial information inherent in phased-array radiofrequency coils to reduce acquisition times. The number of sampled k-space lines can be reduced by a factor of two or more [6]. Now it is possible to image the entire small bowel with fast gradient echo sequences in a single breath-hold using parallel techniques.

There is no consensus on the appropriate protocol, but most studies have performed T2-weighted sequences and contrast-enhanced gradient echo sequences. Parameters vary depending on specific equipment and software available. The author and colleagues routinely perform axial and coronal single-shot sequences throughout the bowel. These sequences are performed during breath-holding. These sequences are susceptible to flow artifacts, and thus intraluminal flow voids can be seen as areas of low signal intensity within the bowel lumen. This appearance can be problematic when one is evaluating for potential intraluminal masses. The administration of glucagon reduces bowel peristalsis and can reduce these artifacts (Fig. 3). The author and colleagues also routinely perform axial and coronal TrueFISP sequences. These sequences can be performed quickly and are complementary to the SSFSE sequences. These sequences also are performed during breath-holding. These sequences demonstrate a black-band artifact at the interface of the bowel wall and mesenteric fat (Fig. 4). This artifact has been described as a potential limitation in assessing bowel wall thickness, but the author and colleagues have not found it a significant limitation. Mesenteric structures are better visualized on the TrueFISP sequence than the single-shot sequence. Mesenteric vessels and lymph nodes are better demonstrated because of the k-space filtering techniques that are performed on single-shot sequences (see Fig. 4). The author and colleagues also obtain a fast gradient echo T1-weighted image through the abdomen before administering intravenous contrast. After administration of intravenous contrast the author and colleagues routinely perform both 2D and 3D gradient echo sequences in a coronal projection followed by 3D axial acquisitions. They routinely use parallel imaging to reduce scan time with the gradient echo sequences. Although the 3D sequences provide better spatial resolution, there is increased image blurring and a decreased signal-to-noise ratio in comparison with the 2D sequences; these limitations may be more noticeable on some of the older platforms (Fig. 5). The appropriate scan delay is yet to be determined. On CT, an enteric phase acquired at approximately 40 to 45 seconds provides peak bowel wall enhancement [28]. A study assessing the use of bowel wall enhancement to diagnose mesenteric ischemia showed that in normal volunteers that the peak wall enhancement for MR imaging occurred during the portal venous phase (at 60–70 seconds) [29]. An advantage of MR imaging is that multiple sequences can be performed repetitively without any concern for ionizing radiation; thus imaging can begin during the enteric phase and continue into the portal venous phase. The

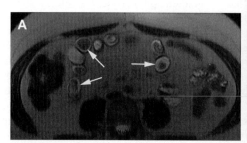
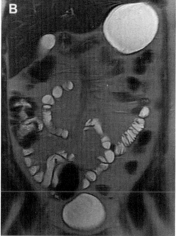

*Fig. 3.* Flow void artifact. (*A*) Axial SSFSE image shows multiple low intensity signal filling defects within small bowel loops (*arrows*) secondary to bowel peristalsis and flow artifacts. (*B*) Coronal SSFSE performed after the administration of glucagon shows a reduction in the flow artifacts.

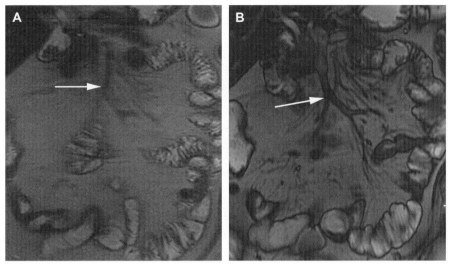

*Fig. 4.* Mesenteric visualization. (*A*) Coronal SSFSE image and (*B*) 2D TrueFISP image. Note the improved conspicuity of the mesenteric structures including mesenteric vessels (*arrows*) and lymph nodes on the TrueFISP sequence. Also note the black-band artifact that occurs at the interface of the bowel wall and mesenteric fat with TrueFISP sequences in panel B.

author and colleagues routinely start imaging approximately 45 seconds after the initiation of contrast injection.

Antiperistaltic agents are critical to improving the quality on the fast gradient echo sequences after intravenous contrast enhancement to reduce bowel peristalsis and blurring (Fig. 6). The author and colleagues administer a split injection of glucagon. They administer 0.5 mg immediately before the initial SSFSE sequences to reduce intraluminal flow voids. They administer a second injection immediately before the injection of intravenous contrast.

## Indications

### *Assessment of Crohn's disease*

Most of the publications using MR to image the small bowel have focused on the imaging of Crohn's disease. Some reports have shown greater than 90% sensitivity and specificity [30,31].

In a previously published study [32], MR enteroclysis showed a sensitivity of 100% in the detection and localization of involved segments, 100% in the identification of wall thickening, 100% in the diagnosis of lumen stenosis and demonstration

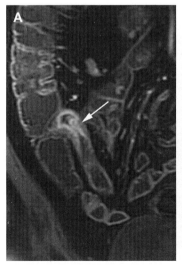
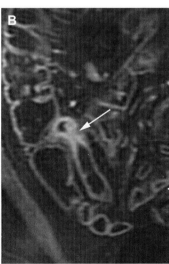

*Fig. 5.* Comparison of 2D and 3D gradient echo sequences. (*A*) Coronal 2D fast spoiled gradient echo image and (*B*) 3D gradient echo image with fat suppression after intravenous administration of contrast shows Crohn's disease in the terminal ileum (*arrow*) with bowel wall thickening, increased mucosal enhancement, and luminal narrowing. Note the slight increase blurring on the 3D gradient echo sequence in panel B.

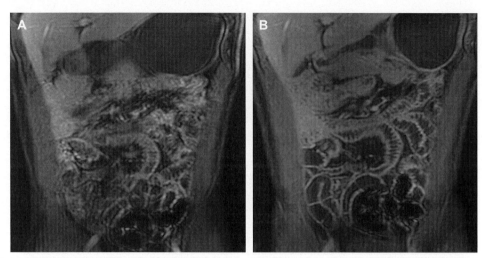

*Fig. 6.* Bowel peristalsis artifact. (*A*) Coronal 2D gradient echo sequence with fat suppression following intravenous administration of contrast without glucagon and (*B*) after administration of glucagon. Note the improved image quality and decreased blurring secondary to peristalsis after glucagon administration in panel B.

of associated prestenotic dilatation, 100% and 88% in the detection of small bowel segments with linear ulcers and superficial lesions, respectively, and 75% in the demonstration of sinus tracts, as compared with conventional enteroclysis. The authors concluded that because the resolution of MR imaging was inferior to that of conventional fluoroscopy, MR enteroclysis may not be indicated for the initial imaging evaluation but has promise in follow-up and assessing complications.

Other studies, some of which have been compared with capsule endoscopy as the criterion, have shown lower sensitivities in the range of 50% to 78% [7,33,34]. In one of these studies MR enterography had a sensitivity of 78% compared with 93% for capsule endoscopy; the difference was not significant ($P > .05$) [33].

Several studies have shown MR imaging to have better sensitivity than barium studies [7,33,35,36]. In a comparison study between conventional enteroclysis and MR enteroclysis, MR enteroclysis demonstrated abnormalities not seen at conventional enteroclysis in 6 of 25 patients (24%). In one of these patients the finding was related to Crohn's disease: MR enteroclysis visualized an ileal fistula, chronic phlegmon, and an abscess that were not detected with conventional enteroclysis. Other findings not detected by conventional enteroclysis but seen on MR imaging included luminal neoplasms and superior mesenteric vein thrombosis [35].

In a study comparing MR enteroclysis with conventional enteroclysis in 27 patients who had Crohn's disease and two patients who had small bowel tumors, MR imaging detected additional findings such as abscesses and fistulas in 20 patients. For the detection of abscesses, with surgery as the criterion, sensitivities were 100% and 0% for MR imaging and conventional enteroclysis, respectively. For the diagnosis of fistula, sensitivity was 83% and 17%, respectively. If visualization of a fistula on either MR imaging or conventional enteroclysis was considered a true-positive result, however, the sensitivity of MR imaging was 84%, and that of conventional enteroclysis was 67% [31].

In a study of active Crohn's disease in the terminal ileum with endoscopy and histology as the criterion, MR enteroclysis had a sensitivity of 89% compared with 72% for conventional enteroclysis. MR imaging detected proximal lesions in nine additional cases not seen by conventional enteroclysis [36].

Only a few published studies have compared CT and MR imaging in the assessment of Crohn's disease. In one study of 26 patients, MR imaging depicted 80% to 85% of abnormal segments, compared with 60% to 65% by CT. Moderate and marked disease was shown equally as well on CT and MR imaging, but for mild disease activity MR imaging detected 68% to 79% of the abnormal segments, compared with 32% to 46% by CT [37]. There was no significant difference in the detection of complication (fistulas, n = 7; phlegmon, n = 3; abscess, n = 3) between MR and CT [37]. In another study, however, investigators found conflicting results. This study compared interobserver agreement and individual sign sensitivity between MR enteroclysis and multidetector CT enteroclysis. These investigators found that there was better interobserver agreement for bowel wall thickening, bowel wall enhancement, and lymphadenopathy on CT enteroclysis than on MR enteroclysis. CT enteroclysis was more sensitive than MR enteroclysis in detecting bowel wall thickening (89% versus 60%), bowel wall enhancement (79% versus 56%), and adenopathy (64% versus 14%) [38]. Therefore, further studies are needed comparing state-of-the-art CT and MR imaging techniques.

The role of MR imaging in assessing colonic inflammation in Crohn's disease has yet to be determined. The author and colleagues routinely perform colonoscopy to map out disease extent in the colon and to evaluate the terminal ileum. Investigators have shown that evaluation of the colon is feasible with MR imaging after the administration of rectal fluid. It also has been shown that the administration of rectal fluid can improve the distention of the distal small bowel loops [12,13,37,39,40]. The author and colleagues have attempted administering rectal fluid in their practice. Patients frequently have difficulty retaining the fluid for the length of the examination. An alternative technique that they have used and that may deserve further investigation is the administration of additional oral contrast over a longer period of time to allow antegrade filling of the colon with fluid (Fig. 7). Patients seem to tolerate this technique better than retrograde filling.

Several findings suggest active inflammation in Crohn's disease and correlate well with acute-phase reactants [27,41,42]. Increased enhancement of the bowel wall is an important finding that is seen with active inflammation (Fig. 8) [27,36]. In a study of 28 patients, gadolinium-enhanced fat-suppressed spoiled gradient-echo sequences had a 96% to 100% per-patient sensitivity in comparison with 60% for unenhanced SSFSE sequences. In addition contrast-enhanced sequences detected more abnormal segments and depicted disease severity more

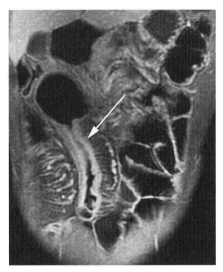

*Fig. 8.* Crohn's disease. Coronal 3D fast gradient echo image with fat suppression after intravenous administration of contrast using enterography technique shows changes of active Crohn's disease consisting of bowel wall thickening, increased mucosal enhancement, luminal narrowing, increased mesenteric vascularity (comb sign), and small bowel obstruction (*arrow*).

correctly than SSFSE sequences [43]. In some mild cases wall enhancement may be seen in the absence of wall thickening, but characterizing disease activity by mild enhancement alone, without any wall thickening on any sequence, can lead to false-positive examinations (Fig. 9).

Several different patterns of enhancement have been described in Crohn's disease. In a study of

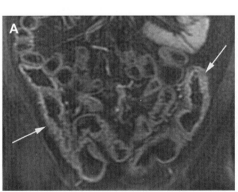
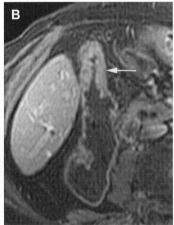

*Fig. 7.* Colonic abnormalities. (*A*) Coronal and (*B*) axial gradient echo images with fat suppression after intravenous administration of contrast performed using enterography technique in two different patients show good antegrade colonic filling with the oral contrast. Note the bowel wall thickening in the colon (*arrows*) in a patient who has ulcerative colitis in panel A and an annular carcinoma (*arrow*) at the hepatic flexure in a different patient in panel B.

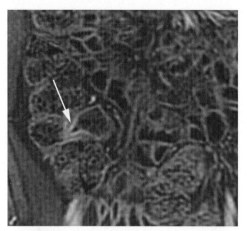

Fig. 9. Crohn's disease. Coronal 3D gradient echo image with fat suppression after intravenous administration of contrast using enterography technique shows subtle area of increased enhancement in the terminal ileum and ileocecal valve (*arrow*) without significant wall thickening. Mild inflammatory changes were noted at colonoscopy and on histology.

58 CT scans, enhancement was classified as type A (multilayered stratification of three or more layers with mucosal and serosal enhancement), type B (two layers with strong mucosal enhancement and low-density submucosa, type C (two layers without

strong mucosal enhancement), and type D (homogenous enhancement) [44]. Ninety-one percent of type A and 100% of type B enhancement patterns had evidence of active inflammation, whereas 86% of type D cases had quiescent disease. Therefore, with active disease the enhancement has a stratified appearance with increased mucosal enhancement, submucosal edema, and, in some cases, serosal enhancement (Fig. 10). This stratified appearance also may suggest that areas of luminal narrowing may respond to medical therapy, whereas areas of wall thickening that are more homogenous and area not stratified or the have low signal intensity on T2-weighted images indicate a more fibrotic or quiescent process that may not respond to medical therapy.

Wall thickening is also usually identified. The normal bowel wall thickness is 3 mm or less. High signal intensity in the bowel wall and surrounding fat can be detected on T2-weighted images and indicates active disease. Fat suppression may improve the conspicuity of the high signal changes in the wall and fat (Fig. 11) [27]. Low signal wall thickening on T2-weighted images with lack of increased enhancement indicates chronic or inactive Crohn's disease.

Deep ulcerations can be identified on both T2-weighted and T1-weighted contrast-enhanced

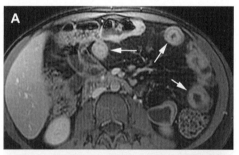

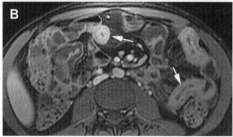

Fig. 10. Crohn's disease. (A and B) Axial 2D fast spoiled gradient echo images with fat suppression after intravenous administration of contrast using enterography technique show stratified appearance of bowel wall enhancement in active Crohn's disease (*arrows*). Note the increased enhancement of the inner mucosal and outer serosal layers with intervening low signal submucosal edema. This appearance implies active inflammatory changes.

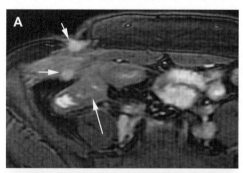

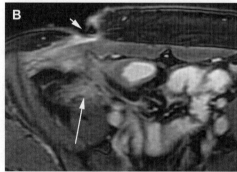

Fig. 11. Crohn's disease. Axial 2D TrueFISP images with fat suppression using enterography technique show (A) high signal intensity wall thickening (*arrow*) and (B) ill-defined high signal phlegmon (*arrow*). Also note the enterocutaneous fistula (*short arrows*) in panels A and B.

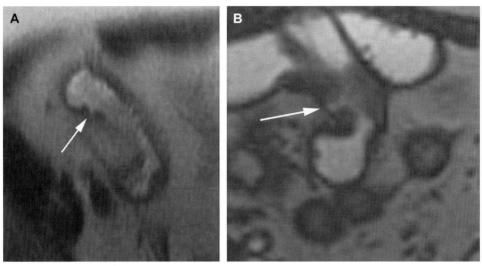

Fig. 12. Crohn's disease ulcer. (*A*) Axial 2D SSFSE and (*B*) TrueFISP images using enterography technique show examples of deep ulcers (*arrows*).

images (Fig. 12). The comb sign indicative of increased blood flow in the vasa recta can be seen in areas of active inflammation (see Fig. 8). The multiplanar capability of MR imaging can demonstrate the asymmetric findings that classically are seen in Crohn's disease (Fig. 13). Other investigators have shown that enhancement of lymph nodes is an important indicator of disease activity [45].

Complications of Crohn's disease include fistulas (see Fig. 11), phlegmons (see Fig. 11), abscesses (see Fig. 2), and bowel obstruction (see Fig. 8).

### Small bowel obstruction

CT has a very high sensitivity for detecting acute, high-grade small bowel obstruction. Because of this sensitivity, and because these examinations can be performed fairly quickly, CT is the main imaging study for this indication. A few studies have shown that MR imaging is capable of detecting small bowel obstruction: two studies that looked at acute small bowel obstructions showed sensitivity of 90% or more [46,47]. In one of these studies, HASTE MR imaging was performed in 43 patients suspected of having small bowel obstruction. MR imaging had 90% sensitivity, with the level of obstruction detected in 73% and the cause in 50%. Obstructing tumors were shown in only three of the six patients. One of the limitations of this study was the lack of intravenous contrast [46]. In another study MR imaging had a sensitivity of 95% and a specificity of 100% in comparison with a sensitivity and specificity of 71% for CT [47].

MR imaging has been shown to have a high sensitivity (90%–93%) for the detection and characterization of malignant versus benign strictures in the

small bowel [48]. In this study 48 patients who had malignancy and bowel obstruction underwent MR imaging. Benign obstruction was seen in 19 cases. Two separate reviewers characterized benign

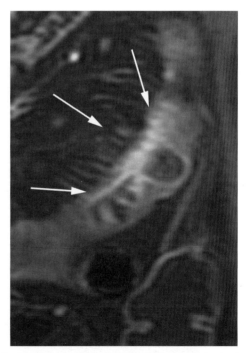

Fig. 13. Crohn's disease. Coronal 3D gradient echo images with fat suppression after intravenous administration of contrast using enterography technique shows classic asymmetric inflammatory changes that occur in Crohn's disease. Note the asymmetric wall thickening, enhancement, and vascularity (*arrows*) along the mesenteric border of the small bowel.

obstruction correctly in 17 and 18 cases, respectively. Malignant obstruction was seen in 29 patients. The reviewers characterized malignant obstruction correctly in 27 and 26 cases, respectively. Features that indicated malignant obstruction included the presence of an obstructing mass, focal or localized segmental mural thickening, and moderate-to-marked peritoneal thickening and enhancement (Fig. 14). Benign obstruction was characterized by the absence of a mass and more generalized or segmental diffuse mural thickening.

Investigators have used MR imaging to map adhesions preoperatively using a visceral slide technique with sensitivity of 87.5% and a specificity of 92.5% [49].

### Small bowel neoplasms

There is a paucity of data comparing the sensitivity of MR imaging and CT and fluoroscopic techniques in the detection of small bowel masses. MR imaging would be useful in routine surveillance of patients who have polyposis syndromes such as Peutz-Jeghers syndrome and familial adenomatous polyposis syndrome, because these patients are at an increased risk for developing small bowel polyps and malignancies and must undergo routine surveillance beginning at a young age. One study compared MR enterography and capsule endoscopy in 20 patients who had polyposis syndromes [50]. Capsule endoscopy detected 448 polyps ranging in size from 1 mm to 30 mm. MR enterography detected only 24 polyps, and all were larger than 5 mm in size. There was no statistically significant difference, however, in the detection rate for larger polyps (> 15 mm), and MR imaging was more accurate in localizing these polyps. These data suggest that MR imaging might be useful for surveillance in patients who have polyposis syndromes. In the author's practice only polyps larger than 1 cm in size are considered for resection to reduce the complications of intussusception or bowel obstruction and the development of malignancy. Further studies would seem indicated to determine if

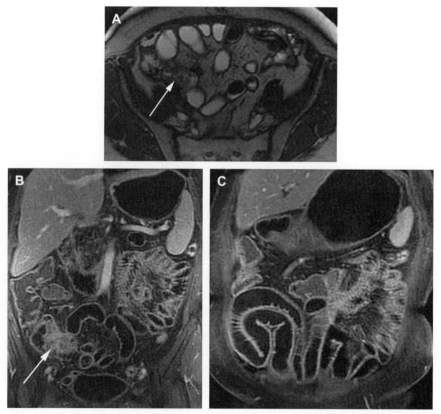

*Fig. 14.* Small bowel obstruction. (*A*) Axial 2D TrueFISP and (*B* and *C*) coronal 2D fast spoiled gradient echo images using enterography technique show focally dilated small bowel loops in the right lower quadrant. A more focal area of bowel wall thickening is also seen in panels A and B. Findings are suggestive of a small bowel obstruction secondary to a mass in this patient who has experienced episodes of chronic low-grade small bowel obstruction. At surgery radiation enteropathy with superimposed lymphoma were discovered.

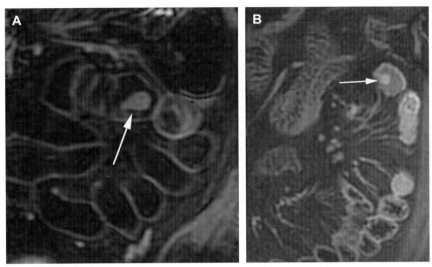

*Fig. 15.* Polyposis syndrome. Coronal 3D gradient echo images with fat suppression after intravenous administration of contrast show small bowel polyps (*arrows*) in two different patients who have (*A*) Peutz-Jegher syndrome (enteroclysis technique) and (*B*) Cowden's syndrome (enterography technique).

state-of-the-art techniques including the use of intravenous contrast can detect polyps larger than 1 cm in size with acceptable accuracy (Fig. 15).

## Summary

Cross-sectional imaging techniques are playing a larger role in the imaging of the small bowel. MR imaging has advantages over CT including the lack of ionizing radiation, improved soft tissue contrast, and the ability to provide real-time and functional evaluation. Limitations that have prevented more widespread implementation of MR imaging in clinical practice include inferior temporal and spatial resolution, access issues, and costs compared with CT. As MR imaging and CT technology continue to advance, further comparative studies will be needed to determine the most accurate technique and their relative advantages to recommend appropriate, cost-effective diagnostic algorithms.

## References

[1] Schwartz DA, Wiersema MJ, Dudiak KM, et al. A comparison of endoscopic ultrasound, magnetic resonance imaging, and exam under anesthesia for evaluation of Crohn's perianal fistulas. Gastroenterology 2001;121(5):1064–72.

[2] Haggett PJ, Moore NR, Shearman JD, et al. Pelvic and perineal complications of Crohn's disease: assessment using magnetic resonance imaging. Gut 1995;36(3):407–10.

[3] Laniado M, Makowiec F, Dammann F, et al. Perianal complications of Crohn disease: MR imaging findings. Eur Radiol 1997;7(7):1035–42.

[4] O'Donovan AN, Somers S, Farrow R, et al. MR imaging of anorectal Crohn disease: a pictorial essay. Radiographics 1997;17(1):101–7.

[5] Froehlich JM, Patak MA, von Weymarn C, et al. Small bowel motility assessment with magnetic resonance imaging. J Magn Reson Imaging 2005; 21(4):370–5.

[6] Glockner JF, Hu HH, Stanley DW, et al. Parallel MR imaging: a user's guide. Radiographics 2005; 25(5):1279–97.

[7] Schreyer AG, Geissler A, Albrich H, et al. Abdominal MRI after enteroclysis or with oral contrast in patients with suspected or proven Crohn's disease. Clin Gastroenterol Hepatol 2004;2(6): 491–7.

[8] Wold PB, Fletcher JG, Johnson CD, et al. Assessment of small bowel Crohn disease: noninvasive peroral CT enterography compared with other imaging methods and endoscopy–feasibility study. Radiology 2003;229(1):275–81.

[9] Rieber A, Aschoff A, Nussle K, et al. MRI in the diagnosis of small bowel disease: use of positive and negative oral contrast media in combination with enteroclysis. Eur Radiol 2000;10(9): 1377–82.

[10] Boraschi P, Braccini G, Gigoni R, et al. MR enteroclysis using iron oxide particles (ferristene) as an endoluminal contrast agent: an open phase III trial. Magn Reson Imaging 2004;22(8): 1085–95.

[11] Laghi A, Paolantonio P, Iafrate F, et al. Oral contrast agents for magnetic resonance imaging of the bowel. Top Magn Reson Imaging 2002; 13(6):389–96.

[12] Herrmann KA, Zech CJ, Michaely HJ, et al. Comprehensive magnetic resonance imaging of the small and large bowel using intraluminal dual contrast technique with iron oxide solution

and water in magnetic resonance enteroclysis. Invest Radiol 2005;40(9):621–9.

[13] Schreyer AG, Golder S, Scheibl K, et al. Dark lumen magnetic resonance enteroclysis in combination with MRI colonography for whole bowel assessment in patients with Crohn's disease: first clinical experience. Inflamm Bowel Dis 2005; 11(4):388–94.

[14] Faber SC, Stehling MK, Holzknecht N, et al. Pathologic conditions in the small bowel: findings at fat-suppressed gadolinium-enhanced MR imaging with an optimized suspension of oral magnetic particles. Radiology 1997;205(1):278–82.

[15] Karantanas AH, Papanikolaou N, Kalef-Ezra J, et al. Blueberry juice used per os in upper abdominal MR imaging: composition and initial clinical data. European Radiology 2000;10(6): 909–13.

[16] Lomas DJ, Graves MJ. Small bowel MRI using water as a contrast medium. Br J Radiol 1999; 72(862):994–7.

[17] Ajaj W, Goehde SC, Schneemann H, et al. Dose optimization of mannitol solution for small bowel distension in MRI. J Magn Reson Imaging 2004;20(4):648–53.

[18] Lauenstein TC, Schneemann H, Vogt FM, et al. Optimization of oral contrast agents for MR imaging of the small bowel. Radiology 2003;228(1): 279–83.

[19] Broglia L, Gigante P, Papi C, et al. Magnetic resonance enteroclysis imaging in Crohn's disease. Radiol Med 2003;106(1–2):28–35.

[20] Laghi A, Carbone I, Paolantonio P, et al. Polyethylene glycol solution as an oral contrast agent for MR imaging of the small bowel. Acad Radiol 2002;2(Suppl 9):S355–6.

[21] Laghi A, Paolantonio P, Catalano C, et al. MR imaging of the small bowel using polyethylene glycol solution as an oral contrast agent in adults and children with celiac disease: preliminary observations. Am J Roentgenol 2003;180(1): 191–4.

[22] Magnano G, Granata C, Barabino A, et al. Polyethylene glycol and contrast-enhanced MRI of Crohn's disease in children: preliminary experience. Pediatr Radiol 2003;33(6):385–91.

[23] Sood RR, Joubert I, Franklin H, et al. Small bowel MRI: comparison of a polyethylene glycol preparation and water as oral contrast media. J Magn Reson Imaging 2002;15(4):401–8.

[24] Borthne AS, Dormagen JB, Gjesdal KI, et al. Bowel MR imaging with oral Gastrografin: an experimental study with healthy volunteers. Eur Radiol 2003;13(1):100–6.

[25] Borthne AS, Abdelnoor M, Hellund JC, et al. MR imaging of the small bowel with increasing concentrations of an oral osmotic agent. Eur Radiol 2005;15(4):666–71.

[26] Papanikolaou N, Prassopoulos P, Grammatikakis J, et al. Optimization of a contrast medium suitable for conventional enteroclysis, MR enteroclysis,

and virtual MR enteroscopy. Abdom Imaging 2002; 27(5):517–22.

[27] Maccioni F, Viscido A, Broglia L, et al. Evaluation of Crohn disease activity with magnetic resonance imaging. Abdom Imaging 2000;25(3): 219–28.

[28] Horton KM, Eng J, Fishman EK. Normal enhancement of the small bowel: evaluation with spiral CT. J Comput Assist Tomogr 2000;24(1): 67–71.

[29] Lauenstein TC, Ajaj W, Narin B, et al. MR imaging of apparent small-bowel perfusion for diagnosing mesenteric ischemia: feasibility study. Radiology 2005;234(2):569–75.

[30] Darbari A, Sena L, Argani P, et al. Gadolinium-enhanced magnetic resonance imaging: a useful radiological tool in diagnosing pediatric IBD. Inflamm Bowel Dis 2004;10(2):67–72.

[31] Rieber A, Wruk D, Potthast S, et al. Diagnostic imaging in Crohn's disease: comparison of magnetic resonance imaging and conventional imaging methods. Int J Colorectal Dis 2000;15(3): 176–81.

[32] Prassopoulos P, Papanikolaou N, Grammatikakis J, et al. MR enteroclysis imaging of Crohn disease. Radiographics 2001;[21 Spec No]:S161–72.

[33] Albert JG, Martiny F, Krummenerl A, et al. Diagnosis of small bowel Crohn's disease: a prospective comparison of capsule endoscopy with magnetic resonance imaging and fluoroscopic enteroclysis. Gut 2005;54(12):1721–7.

[34] Golder SK, Schreyer AG, Endlicher E, et al. Comparison of capsule endoscopy and magnetic resonance (MR) enteroclysis in suspected small bowel disease. Int J Colorectal Dis 2006;21(2): 97–107.

[35] Umschaden HW, Szolar D, Gasser J, et al. Small-bowel disease: comparison of MR enteroclysis images with conventional enteroclysis and surgical findings. Radiology 2000;215(3):717–25.

[36] Ochsenkuhn T, Herrmann K, Schoenberg SO, et al. Crohn disease of the small bowel proximal to the terminal ileum: detection by MR-enteroclysis. Scand J Gastroenterol 2004;39(10): 953–60.

[37] Low RN, Francis IR, Politoske D, et al. Crohn's disease evaluation: comparison of contrast-enhanced MR imaging and single-phase helical CT scanning. J Magn Reson Imaging 2000; 11(2):127–35.

[38] Schmidt S, Lepori D, Meuwly JY, et al. Prospective comparison of MR enteroclysis with multidetector spiral-CT enteroclysis: interobserver agreement and sensitivity by means of "sign-by-sign" correlation. Eur Radiol 2003;13(6): 1303–11.

[39] Ajaj W, Lauenstein TC, Langhorst J, et al. Small bowel hydro-MR imaging for optimized ileocecal distension in Crohn's disease: should an additional rectal enema filling be performed? J Magn Reson Imaging 2005;22(1):92–100.

[40] Narin B, Ajaj W, Gohde S, et al. Combined small and large bowel MR imaging in patients with Crohn's disease: a feasibility study. Eur Radiol 2004;9:1535–42.

[41] Kettritz U, Isaacs K, Warshauer DM, et al. Crohn's disease. Pilot study comparing MRI of the abdomen with clinical evaluation. J Clin Gastroenterol 1995;21(3):249–53.

[42] Sempere GA, Martinez Sanjuan V, Medina Chulia E, et al. MRI evaluation of inflammatory activity in Crohn's disease. AJR Am J Roentgenol 2005;184(6):1829–35.

[43] Low RN, Sebrechts CP, Politoske DA, et al. Crohn disease with endoscopic correlation: single-shot fast spin-echo and gadolinium-enhanced fat-suppressed spoiled gradient-echo MR imaging. Radiology 2002;222(3):652–60.

[44] Choi D, Jin Lee S, Ah Cho Y, et al. Bowel wall thickening in patients with Crohn's disease: CT patterns and correlation with inflammatory activity. Clin Radiol 2003;58(1):68–74.

[45] Gourtsoyiannis N, Papanikolaou N, Grammatikakis J, et al. Assessment of Crohn's disease activity in the small bowel with MR and conventional enteroclysis: preliminary results. Eur Radiol 2004;14(6):1017–24.

[46] Regan F, Beall DP, Bohlman ME, et al. Fast MR imaging and the detection of small-bowel obstruction. AJR Am J Roentgenol 1998;170(6):1465–9.

[47] Beall DP, Fortman BJ, Lawler BC, et al. Imaging bowel obstruction: a comparison between fast magnetic resonance imaging and helical computed tomography. Clin Radiol 2002;57(8):719–24.

[48] Low RN, Chen SC, Barone R. Distinguishing benign from malignant bowel obstruction in patients with malignancy: findings at MR imaging. Radiology 2003;228(1):157–65.

[49] Lienemann A, Sprenger D, Steitz HO, et al. Detection and mapping of intraabdominal adhesions by using functional cine MR imaging: preliminary results. Radiology 2000;217(2):421–5.

[50] Caspari R, von Falkenhausen M, Krautmacher C, et al. Comparison of capsule endoscopy and magnetic resonance imaging for the detection of polyps of the small intestine in patients with familial adenomatous polyposis or with Peutz-Jeghers' syndrome. Endoscopy 2004;36(12):1054–9.

RADIOLOGIC
CLINICS
OF NORTH AMERICA

Radiol Clin N Am 45 (2007) 333–345

ELSEVIER
SAUNDERS

# Virtual Colonoscopy: Technique and Accuracy

Luis A. Landeras, MD[a,b],*, Rizwan Aslam, MBChB[a,b], Judy Yee, MD[a,b]

- Colonic cleansing
  *Sodium phosphate*
  *Magnesium citrate*
  *Polyethylene glycol electrolyte lavage
   solution*
- Colonic distention
  *Spasmolytic agents*

- *Room air*
- *Carbon dioxide*
- Stool and fluid tagging
- Techniques and protocols
- Accuracy
- References

Virtual colonoscopy (VC), also known as CT colonography (CTC), has developed an important role in evaluation of the colon. In some situations it may be a safer method to visualize the colon effectively, or it may be the only available option when other techniques have failed. VC requires the volumetric acquisition of data using helical CT and is ideally achieved with multislice CT technology. Postprocessing of CT data sets is performed on a computer workstation with specific software to generate axial images, multiplanar reformatted views, and three-dimensional (3D) images of the colon. Before the patient is scanned, however, several preparatory steps are required to produce an optimally diagnostic study.

A well-cleansed colon with good distention is essential to achieve a high-quality study for polyp and cancer detection. A poorly prepared colon may be the cause of both false-negative and false-positive findings [1,2]. Standard VC protocol requires scanning the patient in supine and prone positions,

which allows segments of colon with poor cleansing or suboptimal distention in one position to be reevaluated in the opposing position with potentially improved distention and cleansing. The rationale for using various colonic cleansing regimens for VC is discussed. Positive labeling of residual material and electronic subtraction of tagged material are potential strategies to reduce and possibly eliminate the need for purgatives that would further increase patient acceptance of VC compared with other techniques. The two distending agents for VC (room air and carbon dioxide) are discussed, along with practical tips for administration and the role of antispasmodic drugs. A review of state-of-the art VC technique and the results of current performance trials is presented.

## Colonic cleansing

Adequate cleansing of the colon is essential for VC if tagging is not performed. Residual fluid or stool

[a] Department of Radiology, University of California in San Francisco, 505 Parnassus Ave., San Francisco, CA 94143, USA
[b] Department of Radiology, Veterans Affairs Medical Center, 4150 Clement St. (114), San Francisco, CA 94121, USA
* Corresponding author. Department of Radiology, Veterans Affairs Medical Center, 4150 Clement St. (114), San Francisco, CA 94121.
E-mail address: luis.landeras@va.gov (L.A. Landeras).

0033-8389/07/$ – see front matter. Published by Elsevier Inc.
radiologic.theclinics.com

doi:10.1016/j.rcl.2007.03.005

will compromise the diagnostic quality of both two-dimensional (2D) and 3D views [1]. Preparing the bowel for VC consists of two strategies. The first is dietary restriction with little or no solid food consumption and ingestion of clear liquids on the day before the VC scan. The second strategy is the administration of a cathartic agent that promotes evacuation of colonic contents [3].

The preferred laxatives for VC are the saline cathartics such as sodium phosphate and magnesium citrate. These laxatives consist of osmotically active inorganic ions that are not resorbed and remain within the bowel lumen. The osmotic nature of these compounds results in reversal of the normal movement of fluid across the bowel wall, with more fluid entering the bowel lumen than is resorbed. These agents also stimulate peristalsis, resulting in accelerated transit of bowel contents.

### Sodium phosphate

Sodium phosphate is an oral saline cathartic commonly used for bowel cleansing before barium enema examinations and optical colonoscopy. It now is often used for bowel cleansing before VC, and it cleanses the colon effectively. It is known as a "dry prep" because it leaves behind little fluid that could obscure lesions on VC [3,4]. Small particles of residual fecal material that are adherent to the colonic wall may remain, however, and these particles may be mistaken for polyps on VC [1]. Sodium phosphate typically is administered in combination with bisacodyl. Bisacodyl is a contact laxative that acts locally on parasympathetic fibers to induce peristalsis [1]. Multiple studies evaluating cleansing agents for colonoscopy have highlighted better patient compliance with sodium phosphate than with polyethylene glycol (PEG) [5–7]. Studies comparing the efficacy of oral sodium phosphate and PEG electrolyte solution before optical colonoscopy have found no significant difference in the quality of bowel cleansing with these two agents [8–10].

The protocol for the administration of sodium phosphate begins the day before the VC. A single dose (45 mL) of sodium phosphate diluted in 4 oz of water is taken at 6 PM followed by 8 oz of water. This dose is followed by ingestion of four bisacodyl tablets (5-mg each) at 9 PM. A bisacodyl suppository (10 mg) is administered in the morning about 1 hour before leaving for the VC examination. It is important to remind patients to refrain from eating solids and to maintain adequate hydration with clear liquids during this preparatory phase. Ingestion of 8 oz of water is recommended approximately every 2 to 3 hours during the afternoon and evening before the day of the VC examination.

Caution is advised when using sodium phosphate, because it is associated with potential complications related to electrolyte disturbances, such as hyperphosphatemia in up to 39% of patients, hypocalcemia in up to 5% of patients, and hypokalemia and hypernatremia [5,11,12]. Patients who have pre-existing electrolyte abnormalities, renal failure, congestive heart failure, and ascites are particularly at risk and should avoid sodium phosphate [13].

### Magnesium citrate

Magnesium citrate is another saline cathartic that often is used to cleanse the bowel before VC. This agent causes fluid to accumulate in the bowel because of its osmotic effects and promotes peristaltic activity and bowel emptying. Onset of action is usually within 3 hours of ingestion. Although magnesium citrate also has been reported to cause electrolyte imbalances, these changes are less pronounced than those seen with sodium phosphate. Specifically, the marked hyperphosphatemia and hypocalcemia that may result in patients receiving sodium phosphate are not seen with magnesium citrate. Caution is still advised, particularly in patients who have renal insufficiency [14].

Magnesium citrate is available as a premixed solution or in a powder form. The patient ingests 200 to 300 mL (10 ounces) of magnesium citrate the day before the VC examination at approximately 4 PM. A powder form is available containing magnesium carbonate, citric acid, and potassium citrate that the patient mixes with 8 oz of cold water and then ingests. Bisacodyl tablets and suppository are given in addition to magnesium citrate. Four bisacodyl tablets are taken orally with 8 oz of water about 2 hours after drinking the magnesium citrate solutions. A 10-mg bisacodyl suppository is inserted per rectum for final evacuation prior about 1 hour before leaving for the VC scan.

The rationale for this regimen is that the magnesium citrate cleanses the colon, but some residual fluid and stool will remain. The bisacodyl tablets clear the residual material from the proximal colon, and the bisacodyl suppository helps evacuate the distal colon [15]. Magnesium citrate also has been used in conjunction with a decreased volume (2 L) of PEG lavage solution to cleanse the colon before colonoscopy. This technique has been found to reduce preparation time and improve patient tolerance for PEG [16].

### Polyethylene glycol electrolyte lavage solution

Many gastroenterologists prefer PEG electrolyte lavage solution for bowel cleansing before colonoscopy. Patients are required to ingest 4 L of PEG the day before the study. Although PEG is an effective agent for cleansing the bowel, it is not ideal for VC because it often results in excessive retained fluid in the colon and is considered a "wet prep." Excess fluid in the colon limits the diagnostic ability of VC but is not a limitation during optical colonoscopy, because fluid can be removed at the time of the procedure.

Patients often are unable to consume the entire required volume of PEG. In one study 40% of subjects were unable to complete the PEG regimen. In the same study 84% of patients found sodium phosphate to be tolerable, compared with only 33% of patients receiving PEG [17]. Abdominal discomfort, bloating, and nausea and vomiting occur in many patients using PEG. Several studies have found that sodium phosphate is more acceptable to patients than PEG with equivalent levels of colonic cleansing for endoscopic procedures [7–9].

In a study evaluating the effects of two different bowel preparations on residual fluid at VC, 11 patients received PEG and 31 received Phosphosoda. Three reviewers independently assessed the amount of residual colonic fluid in six segments per position per patient. A scoring system was employed in which a score of 1 indicated that no residual fluid remained and 4 indicated that more than 50% of the lumen was filled with fluid. Based on a 12 colonic segmentation pattern (six for supine and six for prone images), a score ranging between 12 and 48 for residual fluid could be obtained. A statistically significant larger amount of fluid was found in the patients who received PEG (mean summed score = 26.91) than in those who received Phosphosoda (mean summed score = 16.30) [18].

## Colonic distention

Adequate distention of the colon is important for obtaining a diagnostic-quality VC examination. Suboptimally distended segments of the colon make polyp and cancer detection difficult, compromising the sensitivity and specificity of the examination. Room air or carbon dioxide may be used for colonic distention for the VC examination. A rectal tube is placed, and approximately 50 to 70 puffs of room air are administered with an insufflation bulb or until the patient experiences fullness or mild discomfort. Although the total colonic volume differs among patients, approximately 2 L of room air is generally sufficient for adequate distention of the entire colon. Alternatively, automatic carbon dioxide insufflation can be used. The electronic carbon dioxide insufflator devices inflate the colon to a maximum preset pressure of 25 mm Hg. The patient then is placed in the supine position, and a scout image of the abdomen and pelvis is acquired. With adequate distention, there will be a complete and full column of gas from the rectum to the cecum. Additional gas may be administered at this stage if the colon is not distended adequately. Once the scan has been performed in the supine position, the patient is placed in the prone position, and another scout image is obtained. Additional gas usually is administered in the prone position to maintain adequate colonic distention. The VC scan then is repeated in the prone position. Scans are performed in dual opposing positions to allow improved distention, particularly of the transverse and sigmoid colon, and also to allow any remaining material in the colon to redistribute (Figs. 1 and 2). Occasionally, limited rescanning is performed with the patient in a decubitus position if there is excess fluid or poor distention of the colon despite these maneuvers. The sigmoid colon usually is the segment of colon that is most difficult to distend adequately. The advantages of scanning subjects in dual opposing positions are well established [19–21]. Yee and colleagues [22] evaluated VC in 182 patients, assessing colonic distention, preparation, and polyp detection data using prone and supine imaging. Colonic distention and preparation were improved significantly by using the two positions in combination. Excellent colonic segmental distention increased when dual position imaging was used (93.7%) as compared with supine (86.4%) or prone (85.6%) imaging alone. The change in position also allowed the displacement of residual fluid and stool, uncovering previously obscured surfaces of the colon (Fig. 3). These results correlated with improved per-patient and per-polyp sensitivity for all polyp sizes.

## Spasmolytic agents

The use of antispasmodic agents such as glucagon or hyoscine butylbromide is controversial. Some radiologists advocate routine use, but many perform VC without the use of spasmolytic agents. The ACR practice guidelines for VC suggest that glucagon can be administered to relieve spasm or patient discomfort.

### Glucagon

Glucagon is a polypeptide hormone that primarily increases blood glucose but also has other actions such as the relaxation of smooth muscle within the gastrointestinal tract. Glucagon has been used widely for its hypotonic effects on the stomach, small intestine, and colon. Many of the published studies evaluating VC for lesion detection have been performed on patients who received 1 mg of glucagon intravenously immediately before scanning. Glucagon acts as a paralytic bowel agent and is thought to improve patient comfort and also to

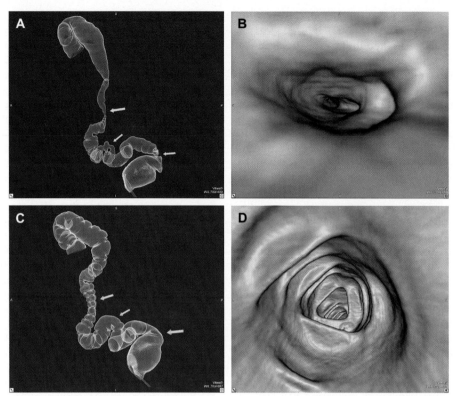

Fig. 1. (*A*) 3D transparent and (*B*) endoluminal images of CT colonography demonstrate inadequate distention of the descending and sigmoid colon (*arrows*). (*C*) 3D transparent and (*D*) endoluminal images in prone position show a well-distended descending and sigmoid colon (*arrows*).

increase colonic distention. Its effect on the bowel varies depending on location. The colon has been found to be the portion of the gastrointestinal tract least sensitive to the effects of glucagon [23]. Adverse reactions to glucagon are relatively uncommon and consist mainly of nausea, vomiting, and headache. Its use is contraindicated in patients who have insulinoma, pheochromocytoma, or poorly controlled diabetes, and in patients who have experienced a previous adverse reaction.

The rationale for using glucagon for VC is based largely on the experience from barium enema studies [24,25]. Thus, it is hoped that glucagon will reduce patient discomfort and improve colonic distention for VC. Rogalla and colleagues [26] performed VC on 240 subjects in the supine position only. The subjects were divided into three groups of 80 each. The first group of 80 received no spasmolytic agent. The other two groups of 80 received glucagon and butyl scopolamine, respectively. The investigators concluded that premedication with butyl scopolamine or, less effectively, glucagon improves colonic distention in the supine position during VC. Yee and colleagues [27] evaluated 60 patients undergoing VC before optical colonoscopy. Thirty-three patients received glucagon immediately before the VC scan, and 27 patients did not. This study showed no significant improvement in colonic distention in patients receiving intravenous glucagon before VC; 444 of 528 segments (84.1%) were adequately distended in the glucagon group, versus 365 of 432 segments (84.5%) in the nonglucagon group. The colonic segments that were most likely to be poorly distended were the descending and sigmoid colon in the supine position and the transverse and sigmoid colon in the prone position; these findings were persistent despite the use of glucagon. One reason for the lack of improved colonic distention despite the use of glucagon may be its effect on the ileocecal valve. Glucagon causes the ileocecal valve to relax, allowing gas to reflux into the small bowel, which then reduces colonic distention. Other studies have found that glucagon does not significantly improve the sensitivity of VC for colorectal polyp detection [28,29].

### Hyoscine butylbromide

Hyoscine butylbromide is an anticholinergic drug that blocks parasympathetic ganglia, causing relaxation of smooth muscle. Although it is not approved for use in the United States, it has been

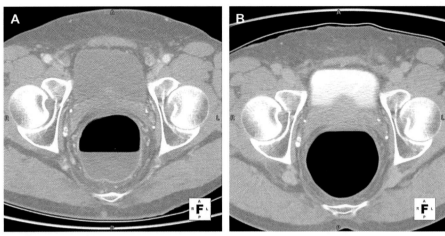

*Fig. 2.* Axial CT images of the colon in the (*A*) supine and (*B*) prone position. The redistribution of fluid with the change in position exposes the whole colonic wall.

used widely in Europe and Asia, where it often is preferred over glucagon as an antispasmodic agent for double-contrast barium enema. Taylor and colleagues [30] performed a study of 136 patients and found that 20 mg hyoscine butylbromide given intravenously significantly improved cecal ($P = .5$), ascending ($P = .001$), and transverse ($P < .001$) colonic distention in the supine position and improved ascending ($P < .001$) and descending ($P < .001$) colonic distention in the prone position. Goei and colleagues [31] directly compared hyoscine butylbromide and glucagon in a study evaluating 324 patients who were referred for double-contrast barium enema. In this study 106 patients received a placebo, 109 patients received 1 mg of intravenous glucagon, and 109 patients received 20 mg of intravenous hyoscine butylbromide before undergoing double-contrast barium enema. Hyoscine butylbromide was found to be more effective than glucagon in distending the colon. One potential drawback highlighted by this study is that approximately 5% of patients who received hyoscine butylbromide experienced blurred vision as a side effect. Other documented side effects of hyoscine butylbromide include tachycardia, dry mouth, acute urinary retention, and acute gastric dilatation. Contraindications to the use of hyoscine butylbromide include glaucoma, obstructive uropathy, gastrointestinal tract obstruction or ileus, severe ulcerative colitis, myasthenia gravis, and unstable cardiac disease.

## Room air

Room air is commonly used for colonic distention during barium enema and optical colonoscopy and also has been widely used for VC largely because of its ease of use, ready availability, and lack of additional cost and because it provides good colonic distention. Room air is composed predominantly of nitrogen, which is poorly absorbed through the colonic wall. Occasionally patients may experience significant abdominal discomfort and pain, particularly after getting off the VC table, and have symptoms for several hours after the VC examination because colonic or small bowel distention persists until the air is expelled distally by peristalsis.

## Carbon dioxide

At some centers carbon dioxide has replaced the use of room air for distention of the colon during VC. One of the main benefits of using carbon dioxide is that it produces negligible postprocedural discomfort and pain. Carbon dioxide is absorbed rapidly through the colonic wall and exhaled through the lungs. Carbon dioxide also has been used for barium enema and optical colonoscopy examinations. Studies have found that pain experienced by patients after a barium enema or VC examination was significantly reduced with carbon dioxide when compared with room air.

In a study of 151 patients, 86 received room air and 65 received carbon dioxide insufflation for double-contrast barium enema. Clinically relevant pain was experienced by 30% of patients after insufflation with room air, compared with only 11% of patients who received carbon dioxide. Five patients reported severe pain after air insufflation. No patients in the carbon dioxide group experienced severe pain [32]. Another study of 142 patients who underwent double-contrast barium enema examination (70 patients received room air and 72 received carbon dioxide) found that carbon dioxide reduced the incidence of immediate and delayed pain from 31% to 12.5% and from 12.9% to 4.2%, respectively [33]. On postevacuation films both studies found more residual colonic

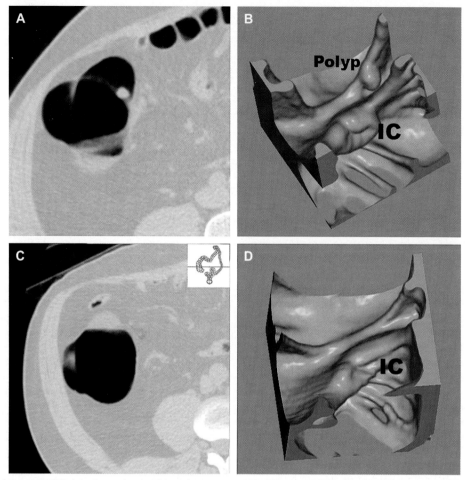

Fig. 3. (*A*) Axial CT image in supine position demonstrates a polyp on a fold. (*B*) 3D cube view clearly demonstrates the polyp. Note close proximity of the ileocecal valve (*IC*). (*C*) Axial CT image in prone position shows redistribution of fluid. No polypoid lesion is identified. (*D*) 3D cube view demonstrates the ileocecal valve (*IC*), and no polypoid lesion is seen.

distention with room air than with carbon dioxide. A recent study by Shinners and colleagues [34] comparing patient-controlled room air with automated carbon dioxide for VC found that carbon dioxide decreased postprocedural discomfort and improved colonic distention.

Other studies evaluating differences in distention have found that the administration of carbon dioxide results in significantly less optimal colonic distention than room air. In a study of 94 patients undergoing barium enema, 49 patients received room air, and 45 patients received carbon dioxide for colonic distention. Patients who received manually administered carbon dioxide had significantly less distention and more mucosal crinkling than patients who received manually administered room air [35]. The problem of poor distention with carbon dioxide seems to have been overcome by the use of automated insufflation of carbon

dioxide. A commercially available electronic insufflation device allows a constant flow of carbon dioxide into the colon per rectum to maintain a preset pressure determined by the user. The maximum pressure setting is at a relatively low level to reduce the risk of colonic rupture. Good colonic distention is maintained during the study, and often, because of the rapid nature of the VC examination, there is little time for significant absorption of carbon dioxide from the colon. Burling and colleagues [36] compared automated and manual insufflation of carbon dioxide in 141 subjects undergoing VC. They found that automated insufflation improved colonic distention overall throughout the colon but particularly in the sigmoid and descending colon when the patients were supine and in the transverse colon when patients were prone, with similar patient acceptance for the two techniques.

## Stool and fluid tagging

Current preparation techniques for VC rely upon rigorous bowel cleansing, which remains a significant limitation of these studies because of patient compliance issues, particularly in the elderly and infirm. Poor patient compliance with the laxative increases the amount of retained material in the colon, causing a significant number of false-positive and false-negative findings. These limitations have prompted research into the possibility of the "prepless" VC using "minimal preparation." In this approach, stool and fluid that remain in the colon are tagged before VC [37–41].

Stool and fluid tagging is performed by the oral administration of barium and/or iodine solution with meals, usually for 24 to 48 h before imaging. This ingestion allows incorporation of the positive contrast material with colonic contents. The high-attenuation tagged stool and residual fluid then are easier to differentiate from the homogenous soft tissue density of polyps (Fig. 4). Once residual stool and fluid are tagged with positive contrast material, electronic subtraction of the high-density material may also be performed (Fig. 5) [42]. It is hoped that the use of tagging will eliminate the need for purgative cleansing of the bowel or at least decrease the amount of laxative required for VC. If significant residual fecal material and fluid are present, and electronic subtraction is unavailable, evaluation of the colonic surface using primary 3D endoluminal assessment will be difficult or impossible to perform.

The American College of Radiology (ACR) practice guideline for performing VC in adults currently does not recommend the routine use of oral contrast for labeling stool or fluid, because this technique is still under evaluation [43]. Several studies, however, have demonstrated promising results (Fig. 6). In a study by Vining [4] of 35 patients who received oral iodinated contrast material 1 to 2 h before the VC, the sensitivity and specificity for detecting polyps larger than 10 mm was reported to be 100% and 85%, respectively. Lefere and colleagues [38] gave 50 patients barium sulfate for fecal tagging, nutritional support, and gentle laxatives and compared polyp detection in these patients with 50 individuals who did not undergo tagging. Results showed 100% sensitivity for polyps measuring 10 mm or larger with no significant difference in sensitivity between tagged and untagged cases. Overall specificity, however, was 11% greater in the tagged group than in controls. Pickhardt and colleagues [40] evaluated 1233 asymptomatic subjects who received tagging before VC. Primary 3D interpretation with electronic subtraction colonography demonstrated higher sensitivity for detection of adenomatous polyps measuring 8 mm or more than with conventional colonoscopy.

In a prospective study using electronically cleansed VC Zalis and colleagues [42] evaluated patient comfort and image readability in 68 subjects who had average-to-moderate risk factors for development of colorectal carcinoma. Tagging techniques included a 2% barium sulfate suspension without cathartics, nonionic iodinated contrast (300 mg/mL) without cathartics, and nonionic iodinated contrast (300 mg/mL) with 34 g of magnesium citrate administered the evening before imaging. Of the three different tagging preparations, the one using a mild cathartic preparation demonstrated the highest subtracted image readability. Readability was defined as little to no discernible unopacified material and artifact as easily interpretable images.

Preliminary studies have also found stool and fluid tagging without the use of cathartics to be feasible [37,44,45]. Lefere and colleagues evaluated 15

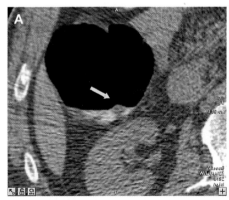
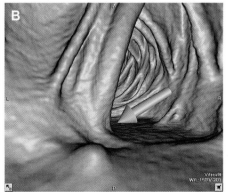

*Fig. 4.* (*A*) Axial image shows a small homogeneous polyp (*arrow*) sitting in a small pool of tagged fluid. (*B*) 3D endoluminal view without subtraction shows the same polyp (*arrow*), which is partially obscured.

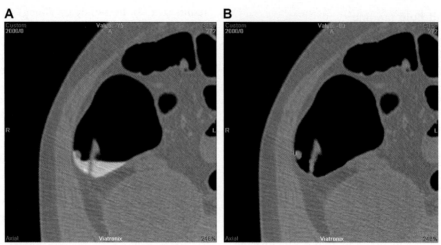

*Fig. 5.* (*A*) Axial CT image in supine position demonstrates a small polyp surrounded by tagged residual fluid. (*B*) Axial CT image after electronic subtraction demonstrates more clearly a small polyp.

patients who underwent VC using a commercially available low-residue diet. Five different tagging regimens were evaluated. The most elaborate tagging protocol started 48 hours prior to scanning with ingestion of 150 mL of a 4% weight per volume (w/v) barium suspension divided in three doses. This was followed by an oral administration of 750 mL of 2.1% w/v barium sulfate the day before examination. The simplest protocol included ingestion of 50 mL total volume of a 40% w/v barium suspension the day prior to VC with regular meals. The amount of liquid ingested was limited to no more than 2 L of fluid the day before VC to yield a balance between ingested fluid and the amount of fluid absorbed in the gastrointestinal tract. This approach allowed a dry colon, so that iodinated contrast material was not required to label residual fluid. Investigators found no significant differences in tagging efficacy among the different barium regimens.

Therefore, the authors preferred the use of 50 mL of a 40% w/v barium suspension administered the day before CTC.

## Techniques and protocols

VC was introduced more than 10 years ago, and since then CT technology has undergone significant advances. State-of-the-art VC requires multidetector CT and a high-end computer workstation with advanced graphic software that displays 2D and 3D views of the colon.

As previously described, patients typically are scanned in a craniocaudal direction in both supine and prone positions. Scanning in the supine and left lateral decubitus positions has been proposed as an alternative to supine and prone scanning whenever patients cannot lie prone. Gryspeerdt and colleagues [46] found improvements in colonic

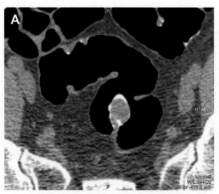
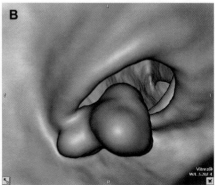

*Fig. 6.* (*A*) Axial image shows a large polyp in the rectum that is surrounded by high-density tagged material. The polyp is homogeneous, and the tagging agent does not penetrate into the lesion, differentiating it from stool. (*B*) Endoluminal image also demonstrates a large polypoid lesion in the rectum.

distention using either supine/prone or supine/left lateral decubitus. Fewer breathing artifacts were noted with left lateral decubitus imaging in elderly patients.

Intravenous contrast material is not administered routinely for screening VC. Disadvantages of the use of intravenous contrast include increased invasiveness, the possibility of contrast reactions, higher radiation dose, increased interpretation times, and higher cost. Intravenous contrast should not be administered if patients undergo oral stool and fluid tagging because of the potential difficulty in differentiating an enhancing lesion from tagged material. Morrin and colleagues [47] found that administration of intravenous contrast significantly improved reader confidence for assessment of bowel wall conspicuity and for the detection of medium-sized polyps (6–9 mm) in suboptimally cleansed colonic segments. When the diagnosis of colon cancer is already established or is suspected based on initial imaging, intravenous contrast should be administered for VC for staging purposes.

A typical VC protocol using multidetector CT consists of a collimation of 0.625 to 2.5 mm with a gantry rotation time of 0.5 seconds resulting in a scan time of less than 10 seconds (Table 1). Multidetector-row CT scanners have enabled subcentimeter collimation without compromising z-axis coverage. The volumetric data set is used for traditional 2D axial images and multiplanar reformats as well as to produce 3D endoluminal views. Motion artifact from peristalsis and respiration is decreased or eliminated with MDCT because scan times are significantly shortened. Several studies have demonstrated that thinner reconstructions allow increased sensitivity for small polyps ($\leq 5$

mm) and improve specificity in both phantom and human datasets [48–51]. Lui and colleagues [48] performed a study in 25 patients and found increased specificity for polyps 5 mm or larger using a slice thickness of 1.25 mm × 1 mm when compared with thicker slices (5 mm × 2 mm) using a four-slice multidetector-row CT.

The ACR practice guidelines for the performance of VC recommend use of multidetector CT with a slice collimation of 3 mm or less and a reconstruction interval of 1.5 mm or less [43]. In a recent consensus study a maximum acceptable slice thickness of 3 mm or less was recommended by 88% (22/25) of selected virtual colonoscopy experts [52].

CTC uses ionizing radiation, and because it has the potential to become a screening test, the effective radiation dose of this examination has been monitored. Because of the intrinsic high contrast between the intraluminal gas and the soft tissue of the colonic wall, dropping the milliampere-second (mAs) can reduce the effective radiation dose to the patient substantially compared with routine CT examinations of the abdomen and pelvis. Macari and colleagues [53] performed VC in 105 subjects using 50 mAs, 120 kilovolt peak (kVp), and a 1.25-mm slice thickness with a 1-mm reconstruction interval. Sensitivity of VC for the detection of polyps 6 to 9 mm and 10 mm or larger were 70% and 93%, respectively. The effective radiation doses for VC were 5.0 millisievert (mSv) for men and 7.8 mSv women. Brenner and Georgsson [54] estimated the absolute lifetime cancer risk associated with radiation exposure using similar parameters to be 0.14% for combined supine and prone VC scans for a 50-year-old person and about half that for a 70-year-old person. Several

**Table 1:** Virtual colonoscopy multidetector CT protocol

| Technical parameters | 16-slice MDCT | 64-slice MDCT |
|---|---|---|
| Respiratory phase | Inspiration | Inspiration |
| Scan area | Entire abdomen and pelvis | Entire abdomen and pelvis |
| Scan direction | Cranial—caudal | Cranial—caudal |
| Scan position | Supine and prone (or lateral decubitus) | Supine and prone (or lateral decubitus) |
| Detector configuration | 16 × 0.625 mm | 64 × 0.625 mm |
| Pitch | 1.375 | 0.984 |
| Feed table (mm/rotation) | 13.75 | 39.4 |
| Gantry rotation time (s) | 0.5 | 0.5 |
| Kilovolt peak (kVp) | 120 | 120 |
| Milliampere (mA)[a,b] | 100 | 100 |
| Reconstruction | Standard/full | Standard/full |
| Thickness (mm) | 1.25 | 1.25 |
| Interval (mm) | 0.8 | 0.8 |

*Abbreviation:* MDCT, multidetector CT.
[a] No x, y tube current modulation is employed.
[b] For larger patients (display field of view > 40 cm), mA value of 200 is used.

investigators have shown that ultra-low-dose VC may be performed using even lower mAs [55–57]. Iannaccone and colleagues [55] compared CTC with optical colonoscopy in 158 patients using 140 kVp, effective mAs of 10, 2.5-mm detector collimation on a four-row multidetector CT. VC depicted all 22 carcinomas and 13 polyps measuring 10 mm or larger (sensitivity = 100%). The effective dose was 1.8 mSv in men and 2.4 mSv in women.

VC has also been demonstrated to be a valuable tool for the identification of extracolonic findings (Fig. 7) [58,59]. In authors' own experience, Yee and colleagues [60] evaluated extracolonic findings in 500 subjects who underwent VC. Clinically important extracolonic findings were identified in 9% of patients (45/500). Currently, screening VC should be performed with a minimum of 50 mAs because lower values probably would preclude optimal evaluation of extracolonic finding [56].

## Accuracy

Multiple single-center studies, including two meta-analyses, and several multicenter trials have demonstrated the ability of CTC to detect colonic-neoplastic lesion,. Mulhall and colleagues [61] performed a meta-analysis of 33 published trials involving 6393 patients with the following inclusion criteria: prospective studies, full bowel preparation, complete colonoscopy or surgery as the criterion standard, at least single-slice helical CT scanner, supine and prone positioning, air or carbon dioxide insufflation, scan interval of 5 mm or less, and use of 2D and 3D views during scan interpretation. The per-patient sensitivity for polyps 10

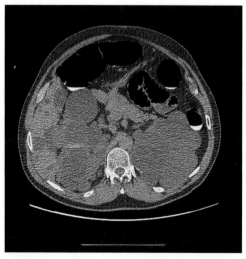

*Fig. 7.* This patient was found to have adult-type polycystic kidney disease when he presented for his CT colonography.

mm or larger, between 6 and 9 mm, and smaller than 6 mm were 85%, 70%, and 48%, respectively. Specificity was 97%, 93%, and 91% for polyps 10 mm or larger, between 6 and 9 mm, and smaller than 6 mm, respectively. A meta-analysis by Halligan and colleagues [62] included 24 studies for a total of 4181 patients. There were similar findings, with a high per-patient average sensitivity of 93% and specificity of 97% for large polyps. High sensitivity (95.9%) also was demonstrated for cancer.

Several large single-center studies have demonstrated high sensitivity and specificity of CTC using single-row or multidetector scanners [21,53,63–65]. Per-polyp sensitivity for medium-sized polyps (6–9 mm) and large polyps (≥10 mm) ranged from 47% to 82% and from 75% to 93%, respectively. Per-patient sensitivity ranged from 76% to 93% for medium-sized polyps and from 84% to 100% for large polyps. Specificity ranged from 88% to 97% for all sizes of polyps.

Three large multicenter trials have been published. Pickhardt and colleagues [40] evaluated a total of 1233 asymptomatic adults who underwent same-day virtual and optical colonoscopy with segmental unblinding. Patients underwent bowel cleansing using a double-dose of sodium phosphate (90 mL) and fecal and fluid tagging using barium and iodinated contrast material. Additionally, primary 3D interpretation with electronic subtraction was performed with 2D views used to evaluate specific potential lesions. Excellent results were achieved: the sensitivity of VC for adenomatous polyps 10 mm and larger, 8 mm and larger and 6 mm and larger was 93.8%, 93.9%, and 88.7%, respectively. The sensitivity of optical colonoscopy for adenomatous polyps was 87.5%, 91.5%, and 92.3%, respectively, for the three sizes of polyps. The specificity of virtual colonoscopy for adenomatous polyps was 96.0%, 92.2%, and 79.6%, respectively, for polyps at least 10 mm, 8 mm, and 6 mm.

Cotton and colleagues [66] evaluated 600 patients who had symptoms of possible colorectal cancer or who had history of polyps. Optical colonoscopy with segmental unblinding was performed. The sensitivity of VC for the detection of polyps 10 mm or larger and 6 to 9 mm was only 52% and 23%, respectively. The sensitivity of optical colonoscopy was 96% and 99%, respectively. Poor results probably were related at least partially to the limited experience of VC readers in eight of the nine centers included in the study. The center with the largest experience in VC reported a sensitivity of 82% for lesions larger than 6 mm.

Rockey and colleagues [67] demonstrated similar disappointing results in a study of 614 patients at increased risk for colorectal cancer. All patients underwent air-contrast barium enema (ABCE), CTC, and optical colonoscopy with segmental unblinding. The sensitivity for detecting lesions 10 mm or larger was 45% for ACBE, 53% for VC, and 99% for colonoscopy. For lesions 6 to 9 mm in size the sensitivity of ACBE was 30%, compared with 47% for VC and 99% for colonoscopy. Half of the readers had experience reading more than 50 VC examinations. VC readers with less experience were asked to complete a VC training module, although no testing was performed. The ACR Imaging Network (ACRIN) National CT Colonography trial (#6664) is now underway with a total expected recruitment of 2607 subjects (www.acrin.org). This is a multicenter trial evaluating the performance of VC in a large screening patient cohort including 15 sites. It is expected to address issues related to interpretation methods, stool and fluid tagging, and second reads. A database of cases will be created for further evaluation of CTC including computer-aided detection.

VC continues to evolve as a less invasive tool for evaluation of the colon in both diagnostic and screening settings. The accuracy of this examination depends on adequate patient cleansing and distention, optimal CT technique, and interpretation by a trained reader. The potential benefit of CTC, particularly in a screening population, is large, and it is already changing the way the colon is evaluated.

## References

[1] Yee J. CT colonography: examination prerequisites. Abdom Imaging 2002;27(3):244–52.

[2] Fletcher JG, Johnson CD, MacCarty RL, et al. CT colonography: potential pitfalls and problem-solving techniques. AJR Am J Roentgenol 1999; 172(5):1271–8.

[3] Gelfand DW, Chen MYM, Ott DJ. Preparing the colon for the barium enema examination. Radiology 1991;178(3):609–13.

[4] Vining DJ. Optimizing bowel preparation. In: Book of abstracts. First International Symposium on Virtual Colonoscopy 1998. Boston: Boston University Press. p. 79–80.

[5] Mathus-Vliegen EM, Kemble UM. A prospective randomized blinded comparison of sodium phosphate and polyethylene glycol-electrolyte solution for safe bowel cleansing. Aliment Pharmacol Ther 2006;23(4):543–52.

[6] Vanner SJ, Macdonald PH, Paterson WG, et al. A randomized prospective trial comparing oral sodium phosphate with standard polyethylene glycol based lavage solution (Golytely) in the preparations of patients for colonoscopy. Am J Gastroenterol 1990;85(4):422–7.

[7] Frommer D. Cleansing ability and tolerance of three bowel preparations for colonoscopy. Dis Colon Rectum 1997;40(1):100–4.

[8] Marshall JB, Pineda JJ, Barthel JS, et al. Prospective, randomized trail comparing sodium phosphate solution with polyethylene glycol-electrolyte lavage for colonoscopy preparation. Gastrointest Endosc 1993;39(5):631–4.

[9] Afridi SA, Barthel JS, King PD, et al. Prospective, randomized trial comparing a new sodium phosphate-bisacodyl regimen with conventional PEG-ES lavage for outpatient colonoscopy preparation. Gastrointest Endosc 1995;41(5):485–9.

[10] Arezzo A. Prospective randomized trial comparing bowel cleaning preparations for colonoscopy. Surg Laparosc Endosc Percutan Tech 2000; 10(4):215–7.

[11] Ehrenpreis ED, Nogueras JJ, Botoman VA, et al. Serum electrolyte abnormalities secondary to Fleet's Phospho-Soda colonoscopy prep. Surg Endosc 1996;10(10):1022–4.

[12] Vukasin P, Weston LA, Beart RW. Oral Fleet Phospho-Soda laxative-induced hyperphosphatemia and hypocalcemic tetany in an adult: report of a case. Dis Colon Rectum 1997;40(4):497–9.

[13] Fass R, Do S, Hixson LJ. Fatal hyperphosphatemia following Fleet Phospho-Soda in a patient with colonic ileus. Am J Gastroenterol 1993; 88(6):929–32.

[14] Wiberg JJ, Turner GG, Nuttall FQ. Effect of phosphate or magnesium cathartics on serum calcium: observations in normocalcemic patients. Arch Intern Med 1978;138(7):1114–6.

[15] Bartram CI. Bowel preparation—principles and practice. Clin Radiol 1994;49(6):365–7.

[16] Sharma VK, Chockalingham SK, Ugheoke EA, et al. Prospective, randomized, controlled comparison of the use of polyethylene glycol electrolyte lavage solution in four-liter versus two-liter volumes and pretreatment with either magnesium citrate or bisacodyl for colonoscopy preparation. Gastrointest Endosc 1998;47(2):167–71.

[17] Hookey LC, Depew WT, Vanner SJ. A prospective randomized trial comparing low-dose oral sodium phosphate plus stimulant laxatives with large volume polyethylene glycol solution for colon cleansing. Am J Gastroenterol 2004;99(11): 2217–22.

[18] Macari M, Lavelle M, Pedrosa I, et al. Effect of different bowel preparations on residual fluid at CT colonography. Radiology 2001;218(1):274–7.

[19] Chen SC, Lu DS, Hecht JR, et al. CT colonography: value of scanning in both the supine and prone positions. AJR Am J Roentgenol 1999; 172(3):595–9.

[20] Morrin MM, Farrell RJ, Keogan MT, et al. CT colonography: colonic distention improved by dual positioning but not intravenous glucagon. Eur Radiol 2002;12(3):525–30.

[21] Fletcher JG, Johnson CD, Welch TJ, et al. Optimization of CT colonography technique: prospective trial in 180 patients. Radiology 2000; 216(3):704–11.

[22] Yee J, Kumar NN, Hung RK, et al. Comparison of supine and prone scanning separately and in combination at CT colonography. Radiology 2003;226(3):653–61.

[23] Chernish SM, Maglinte DD. Glucagon: common untoward reactions review and recommendations. Radiology 1990;177(1):145–6.

[24] Meeroff JC, Jorgens J, Isenberg JI. The effect of glucagon on barium enema examination. Radiology 1975;115(1):5–7.

[25] Bova JG, Jurdi RA, Bennett WF. Antispasmodic drugs to reduce discomfort and colonic spasm during barium enemas: comparison of oral hyoscyamine, i.v. glucagon, and no drug. AJR Am J Roentgenol 1993;161(5):965–8.

[26] Rogalla P, Lembcke A, Rückert JC, et al. Spasmolysis at CT colonography: butyl scopolamine versus glucagon. Radiology 2005;236(1):184–8.

[27] Yee J, Hung RK, Akerkar GA, et al. The usefulness of glucagon hydrochloride for colonic distention in CT colonography AJR Am J Roentgenol 1999;173(1):169–72.

[28] Yee J, Hung RK, Steinauer-Gebauer AM, et al. Colonic distention and prospective evaluation of colorectal polyp detection with and without glucagon during CT colonography [abstract]. Radiological Society of North America Scientific Program 1999;213(Suppl):256.

[29] Morrin MM, Kruskal JB, Farrell RJ, et al. Does glucagon improve colonic distention and polyp detection during CT colonography [abstract]. Radiological Society of North America Scientific Program 1999;213(Suppl):341.

[30] Taylor SA, Halligan S, Goh V, et al. Optimizing colonic distention for multi-detector row CT colonography: effect of hyoscine butylbromide and rectal balloon catheter. Radiology 2003;229(1):99–108.

[31] Goei R, Nix M, Kessels AH, et al. Use of antispasmodic drugs in double contrast barium enema examination: glucagon or Buscopan? Clin Radiol 1995;50(8):553–7.

[32] Coblentz CL, Frost RA, Molinaro V, et al. Pain after barium enema: effect of $CO_2$ and air on double-contrast study. Radiology 1985;157(1):35–6.

[33] Robson NK, Lloyd M, Regan F. The use of carbon dioxide as an insufflation agent in barium enema—does it have a role? Br J Radiol 1993;66(783):197–8.

[34] Shinners TJ, Pickhardt PJ, Taylor AJ, et al. Patient-controlled room air insufflation versus automated carbon dioxide delivery for CT colonography. AJR Am J Roentgenol 2006;186(6):1491–6.

[35] Scullion DA, Wetton CWN, Davies C, et al. The use of air or $CO_2$ as insufflation agents for double contrast barium enema (DCBE): is there a qualitative difference? Clin Radiol 1995;50(8):558–61.

[36] Burling D, Taylor SA, Halligan S, et al. Automated insufflation of carbon dioxide for MDCT colonography: distension and patient experience compared with manual insufflation. AJR Am J Roentgenol 2006;186(1):96–103.

[37] Callstrom MR, Johnson CD, Fletcher JG, et al. CT colonography without cathartic preparation: feasibility study. Radiology 2001;219(3):693–8.

[38] Lefere PA, Gryspeerdt SS, Dewyspelaere J, et al. Dietary fecal tagging as a cleansing method before CT colonography: initial results—polyp detection and patient acceptance. Radiology 2002;224(2):393–403.

[39] Zalis ME, Hahn PF. Digital subtraction bowel cleansing in CT colonography. AJR Am J Roentgenol 2002;176:646–8.

[40] Pickhardt PJ, Choi JR, Hwang I, et al. Computed tomographic virtual colonoscopy to screen for colorectal neoplasia in asymptomatic adults. N Engl J Med 2003;349(23):2191–200.

[41] Zalis ME, Perumpillichira JJ, Kim JY, et al. Polyp size at CT colonography after electronic subtraction cleansing in an anthropomorphic colon phantom. Radiology 2005;236(1):118–24.

[42] Zalis ME, Perumpillichira JJ, Magee C, et al. Tagging-based, electronically cleansed CT colonography: evaluation of patient comfort and image readability. Radiology 2006;239:149–59.

[43] American College of Radiology. ACR practice guideline for the performance of computed tomography (CT) colonography in adults. Reaston (VA): American College of Radiology; 2005. p. 295–9.

[44] Iannaccone R, Laghi A, Catalano C, et al. Computed tomographic colonography without cathartic preparation for the detection of colorectal polyps. Gastroenterology 2004;127(5):1300–11.

[45] Lefere P, Gryspeerdt S, Baekelandt M, et al. Laxative-free CT colonography. AJR Am J Roentgenol 2004;183(4):945–8.

[46] Gryspeerdt SS, Herman MJ, Baekelandt MA, et al. Supine/left decubitus scanning: a valuable alternative to supine/prone scanning in CT colonography. Eur Radiol 2004;14(5):768–77.

[47] Morrin MM, Farrell RJ, Kruskal JB, et al. Utility of intravenously administered contrast material at CT colonography. Radiology 2000;217(3):765–71.

[48] Lui YW, Macari M, Israel G, et al. CT Colonography data interpretation: effect of different section thicknesses—preliminary observations. Radiology 2003;229:791–7.

[49] Chung DJ, Huh KC, Choi WJ, et al. CT colonography using 16-MDCT in the evaluation of colorectal cancer. AJR Am J Roentgenol 2005;184(1):98–103.

[50] Laghi A, Iannaccone R, Mangiapane F, et al. Experimental colonic phantom for the evaluation of the optimal scanning technique for CT colonography using a multidetector spiral CT equipment. Eur Radiol 2003;13:459–66.

[51] Won HJ, Choi BI, Kim SH, et al. Protocol optimization of multidetector computed tomography colonography using pig colonic phantoms. Invest Radiol 2005;40(1):27–32.

[52] Barish MA, Soto JA, Ferrucci JT. Consensus on current clinical practice of virtual colonoscopy. AJR Am J Roentgenol 2005;184:786–92.

[53] Macari M, Bini EJ, Xue X, et al. Colorectal neoplasms: prospective comparison of thin section low-dose multi-detector row CT colonography and conventional colonoscopy for detection. Radiology 2002;224(2):383–92.

[54] Brenner DJ, Georgsson MA. Mass screening with CT colonography: should the radiation exposure be of concern? Gastroenterology 2005;129:328–37.

[55] Iannaccone R, Laghi A, Catalano C, et al. Detection of colorectal lesions: lower-dose multi-detector row helical CT colonography compared with conventional colonoscopy. Radiology 2003;229(3):775–81.

[56] van Gelder RE, Venema HW, Serlie IW, et al. CT colonography at different radiation dose levels: feasibility of dose reduction. Radiology 2002;224(1):25–33.

[57] van Gelder RE, Venema HW, Florie J, et al. CT colonography: feasibility of substantial dose reduction—comparison of medium to very low doses in identical patients. Radiology 2004;232(2):611–20.

[58] Hara AK, Johnson CD, MacCarty RL, et al. Incidental extracolonic findings at CT colonography. Radiology 2000;215:353–7.

[59] Rajapksa RC, Macari M, Bini EJ. Prevalence and impact of extracolonic findings in patients undergoing CT colonography. J Clin Gastroenterol 2004;38:767–71.

[60] Yee J, Kumar NN, Godara S, et al. Extracolonic abnormalities discovered incidentally at CT colonography in a male population. Radiology 2005;236(2):519–26.

[61] Mulhall BP, Veerappan GR, Jackson JL. Meta-analysis: computed tomographic colonography. Ann Intern Med 2005;142(8):635–50.

[62] Halligan S, Altman DG, Taylor SA, et al. CT colonography in the detection of colorectal polyps and cancer: systematic review, meta-analysis, and proposed minimum data set for study level reporting. Radiology 2005;237(3):893–904.

[63] Yee J, Akerkar GA, Hung RK, et al. Colorectal neoplasia: performance character after colonography detection in 300 patients. Radiology 2001;219:685–92.

[64] van Gelder R, Yung Nio C, Florie J, et al. Computed tomographic colonography compared with colonoscopy in patients at increased risk for colorectal cancer. Gastroenterology 2004;127(1):41–8.

[65] Hara A, Johnson CD, Welch TJ, et al. CT colonography: single- versus multi-detector row imaging. Radiology 2001;219:461–5.

[66] Cotton PB, Durkalski VL, Pineau BC, et al. Computed tomographic colonography (virtual colonoscopy): a multicenter comparison with standard colonoscopy for detection of colorectal neoplasia. JAMA 2004;291(14):1713–7.

[67] Rockey DC, Paulson R, Niedzwiecki D, et al. Analysis of air contrast barium enema, computed tomographic colonography, and colonoscopy: prospective comparison. Lancet 2005;363(9456):305–11.

RADIOLOGIC
CLINICS
OF NORTH AMERICA

Radiol Clin N Am 45 (2007) 347–359

# CT Colonography: Visualization Methods, Interpretation, and Pitfalls

Abraham H. Dachman, MD, FACR[a],*, Philippe Lefere, MD[b],
Stefaan Gryspeerdt, MD[b], Martina Morin, MD, FFRRCSI, FRCR[c]

- Visualization and interpretation methods
  *Two-dimensional visualization and
    interpretation*
  *Three-dimensional endoluminal
    visualization and interpretation*
  *Bells and whistles*

- *Novel views*
- Common pitfalls in virtual colonoscopy
- Summary
- Acknowledgments
- Appendix 1
- References

## Visualization and interpretation methods

Interpretation of CT colonography (CTC) often involves three-dimensional (3D) visualization using specialized software developed for this application as an adjunct or alternative to conventional two-dimensional (2D) multiplanar reconstruction (MPR) visualization. There is debate as to the relative value of 2D versus 3D for primary interpretation of CTC [1]. This controversy extends to novel displays that flatten the open colon and other innovative viewing methods [2–7]. The 2D-versus-3D controversy is important because it may influence the ease of interpretation for novice readers and the learning curve in CTC interpretation. Differences in software can impact the use of computer-aided detection (CAD) of polyps and novel reading tools such as semiautomated comparison of supine and prone positioning, measurements of polyp size and volume, and recognition of pitfalls of

interpretation. This article presents some of the old and new visualization packages as well as cutting-edge software, some of which is still undergoing improvements and innovations. The authors illustrate several methods without expressing their own preferences. Some pitfalls of CTC interpretation are identified. Because many readers of this article will not have had personal experience with CTC, it is important to appreciate that only a full hands-on review of a software program should be used when making purchasing decisions. This article may serve as a guide to identify features of specific CTC visualization tools. For the reader's convenience, the URL links of common software vendors are listed in Appendix 1.

No visualization program can compensate for a poorly executed CTC examination. If the colon is poorly distended, poorly cleansed, or, in the case of "prepless" CTC, residual fluid or stool is poorly tagged with oral contrast agents, the

Dr. Dachman is a consultant to EZ-E-EM, Inc., GE Healthcare, Inc., Philips Medical Systems, Inc,m and iCAD, Inc. and has research support from iCAD, Inc.

[a] Department of Radiology, MC2026, The University of Chicago, 5841 S. Maryland Ave., Chicago, IL 60645, USA
[b] Department of Radiology, Stedelijk Ziekenhuis, Bruggesteenweg 90, B-8800 Roeselare, Belgium
[c] Department of Radiology, Beaumont Hospital, Beaumont Road, Dublin 9, Ireland
* Corresponding author.
*E-mail address:* ahdachma@uchicago.edu (A.H. Dachman).

doi:10.1016/j.rcl.2007.03.007

interpretation will be either impossible or extremely difficult. The authors emphasize the need for both good training and technique in performing CTC examinations [8].

Several experts believe that the 2D-versus-3D controversy is exaggerated in the literature. In practice, it is critical to have good reading skills in both 2D and 3D. A primary 2D interpretation requires 3D problem solving, and vice versa [9–11]. 2D skills, however, are more difficult to acquire (especially for a radiologist not accustomed to abdominal imaging) and maintain. Nonradiologists find 2D skills particularly difficult. These skills are critical in detecting flat lesions [12], distinguishing stool from polyps, and evaluating pitfalls such as colonic mobility that cause the reader to misinterpret a real polyp as mobile stool [13,14]. These pitfalls are outlined in greater detail later. 3D reading, which often refers to a primary endoluminal perspective fly-though, is more intuitive and less fatiguing. Some pitfalls are unique to particular viewing software, such as artifacts created by electronic subtraction on 3D images. Thus the issues of viewing methods and pitfalls are related topics, and both are discussed.

## Two-dimensional visualization and interpretation

The critical elements of any CTC 2D visualization software are the ease of comparing different images by simultaneously viewing and of making point-to-point correlation between images (Box 1). These include

1. Comparison of supine and prone images with the option of linking images at the same level
2. Comparison of any choice of MPRs (axial, coronal, sagittal, oblique) with linking of source supine and prone images
3. Comparison of various window/level settings with presets for lung, soft tissue, and intermediate (wide soft tissue window for detecting flat lesions)
4. Independent window/level settings for any single view when multiple views are displayed

An example showing simultaneous supine and prone comparison with axial and coronal comparisons is shown in Fig. 1. Adjustable linking of supine and prone views facilitates comparison and problem solving.

To clarify the importance of the fourth point, if one were using stool and fluid tagging, particularly with a mild cathartic preparation or without any cathartic, it is valuable to view the same image in a wide "bone" window (Fig. 2) to see if any polyps were enveloped by the residual tagged stool, while

---

**Box 1:   Features for CTC software**

*Basic features*
Comparison of supine and prone positioning with locking feature
Axial-to-multiplanar comparison
Magnification and image roam
Independent magnification of only selected views
Interactive window/level
Surface- or volume-rendered endoluminal views
Lower threshold adjustment if surface rendered
Comparison of 2D to endoluminal views, and vice versa
Point-to-point pixel comparison, 2D to 3D views, and vice versa
Measuring tools on 2D and 3D
Highly reliable colon segmentations and removal of noncolon structures
3D overview of segmented colon (solid or transparency view)
Automatic centerline for endoluminal view
Automatic 3D fly-through features with manual navigation options
User-selected viewing angle and fly speed in 3D endoluminal view

*Advanced or features[a]*
Automatic polyp detection (CAD)
High-quality false-positive reduction for CAD
Electronic subtraction of tagged fluid
Electronic subtraction of solid tagged stool
Color maps of CT density on 3D views
Automatic polyp size measurement
Automatic polyp volume measurement
Anatomic features to match supine to prone position reliably
Distance of polyp location from anal verge
Cut open view of colon (several types)
Cut open view of colon without morphing
Integration of all applicable features with novel views (eg, CAD, point-to-point comparisons)
Automatic reporting and photographing tools
Integration of CT colonography reporting and data system scheme to reporting tools

Generic descriptions are used to avoid manufacturer-specific nomenclature
[a] Some of these features are available, and some are under development. The user should be able to turn these features on or off as necessary. All automatic features should permit the user to verify and correct measurements or start/end points when applicable.

---

simultaneously viewing lung windows of the same image.

Other layouts provide more choices by using either dual monitors or smaller images displayed

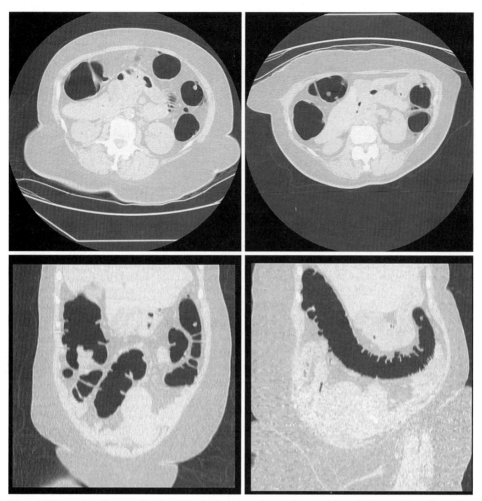

*Fig. 1.* **Primary 2D reading layout simultaneously showing the supine position (*left panels*) and prone position (*right panels*) with the upper row in the axial plane and lower row in the coronal plane. Any viewing box can be changed to any type of view (MPR or 3D) using a pull-down menu.**

on one monitor in a 4-, 5-, or 6-on-1 layout. These approaches permit comparison of 2D images and 3D images of various types at the same time.

### Three-dimensional endoluminal visualization and interpretation

The classic 3D endoluminal view is either surface or volume rendered. All user-friendly software programs should perform a highly accurate segmentation of the colon and eliminate other gas-containing structures such as stomach, small intestines, and the lung bases. The software also should be able to deal with collapsed segments by allowing the user to bridge collapsed segments. No software program is infallible, and therefore there must be a user interface to permit the reader to verify the accuracy of the segmentation of the colon and the bridging of collapsed segments.

Likewise, all good programs should have a high-quality automated centerline and the ability to fly through the colon at a variable speed or to fly through the colon manually. The reader should be able to stop the fly-though at any point and manipulate the viewing direction and the viewing angle. Not all programs are equally user-friendly in performing these basic functions. It should be easy to do point-to-point correlation from the 3D images to the 2D images to determine whether any polyp candidate candidate is stool or soft tissue. Polyp-measuring tools should work well in 3D.

For both surface- and volume-rendered images, the user should know how to optimize the viewing parameters permitted by the software. Some programs allow users to vary these parameters; others do not. For example, in the case of surface-rendered views, many "floaters" within the lumen are seen when the scan is "photon starved," meaning the

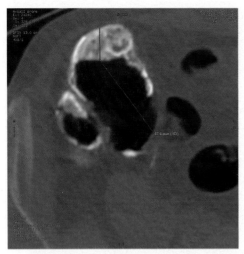

Fig. 2. Prepless virtual colonoscopy with stool tagging. A window of 5000 Hu and level of 900 Hu are used here to view densely tagged stool and fluid. The height of the fluid level is measured at 17.4 mm within which are several particulate pieces of stool characterized by both high-density tagging agent (barium) and low-density gas and fat.

mAs is low relative to the body, as often occurs in the pelvis. The surface-rendered view can be improved by raising the lower-end threshold. In addition, other parameters such as "lighting" and "viewing angle" can be changed.

Some vendors offer a 3D cube in which the cutting plane, magnification, and viewing angle can be altered for 3D problem solving (Fig. 3). This cube shows the inner surface of the colonic wall and can be turned in all directions. Dragging with the mouse allows the reader to enlarge or diminish

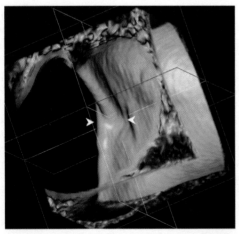

Fig. 3. Cube view for problem solving allows easy manipulation of viewing angle and cutting plane of any 3D image. This technique is helpful when a finding on 2D requires 3D investigation of a single target lesion.

the cube, allowing better localization and visualization of the region of interest.

For a primary 2D reading, the ability to compare 2D with 3D images in a user-friendly manner (preferably with one mouse click) is mandatory. When the reader clicks on a region of interest on the 2D image, the corresponding 3D view should be displayed, allowing inspection in all directions. The point-of-interest view shows a cube of tissue surrounding the region where 3D problem solving is necessary.

### Bells and whistles

Several software programs assist in generating reports by using pull-down menus and tools to help record key images (see Box 1). The distance of the polyp from the rectum also can be obtained automatically to assist the endoscopist or surgeon in finding the polyp or mass.

Electronic subtraction (Fig. 4) [15] of opacified fluid and stool, when sufficiently dense, can help optimize a primary 3D reading, and software with this feature soon will be released by several vendors. Electronic subtraction may cause artifacts on the 2D view, which usually can be easily recognized but are annoying to novice readers.

Up to 20% of the colonic mucosa may be obscured on a unidirectional fly-through [16]. It might be useful to see which areas were not within the view of the virtual camera so one can pay closer attention to them by flying though in the opposite direction and/or viewing the region in 2D. Some software programs can colorize the mucosal surfaces that were not within the line of sight of the virtual camera (Fig. 5).

A problem of primary 3D reading is that each piece of solid stool (both tagged and nontagged) produces a pseudopolypoidal image. Stool can be identified by its texture on 2D views. In a 3D reading, however, it may be convenient to resolve the question of polyp versus stool by using a color map (eg, "Transparency Rendering", Viatronix Inc., Stony Brook, New York) [17] that helps distinguish stool from a fold (Fig. 6).

Automated measurements of polyps can help find the longest dimension of a polyp, as recommended by the Boston Working Group [18]. This information can help optimize size measurements for polyps that are not perfectly hemispherical. Oval and irregularly shaped polyps are probably best measured on the 3D endoluminal views when the polyp can be viewed from several angles before the reader decides how best to measure the lesion. Nevertheless, the reader should confirm the automated measurement before using it to report the case. This precaution is particularly important for polyps 5 to 9 mm in size, because a few millimeters

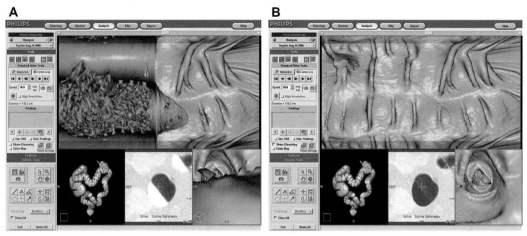

Fig. 4. Electronic subtraction with a filet view workstation layout showing Filet View (which appears to "cut the colon open" and lay it flat, showing one short segment at a time in a movie loop fashion) in the upper panel and 2D view in the lower middle panel (A) without and (B) with electronic subtraction of tagged fluid. The tagged fluid is white in the 2D view and produces a bizarre artifact on the right aspect of the associated filet view (viewer's left). (Courtesy of Philips Medical Systems, Inc., Bothell, WA; with permission.)

difference could change patient management from an immediate colonoscopy to a follow-up CTC.

Polyp volume is a potential new metric for evaluating the change in a polyp over time when comparing two examinations in the same patient [19]. Further research is needed to compare this metric to the traditional measurement of polyp size based on longest dimension.

Semiautomated comparison of supine and prone views is also a tool developed by some researchers to aid in comparing views (Fig. 7) [20]. When a possible polyp is found on one view, and it appears solid (lacking the heterogeneity of stool) and does not seem to be a fold (based on comparison of 2D and 3D views), the next step is to compare the supine and prone views to see if the polyp candidate moved. (If it is mobile, it is important to ensure that there is no stalk and that there is no colonic mobility mimicking the mobility of stool). Currently, the point-to-point comparison between supine and prone views is a skill that novice readers find difficult. This comparison is aided by comparing an overview of the whole colon as seen on 3D transparency or volume-rendered views (simulating a barium enema) or by paging through coronal views. If the computer could help localize the point-to-point comparison of the two series, this would be a particularly helpful tool.

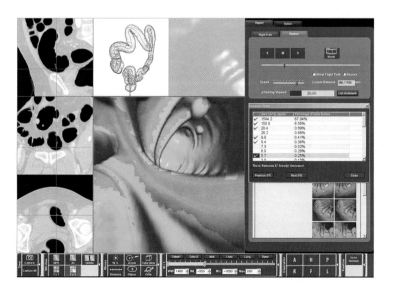

Fig. 5. Paint feature: a workstation layout of one vendor showing lower middle panel in paint mode. The green areas represent colonic surface not seen on one unidirectional fly-through. (Courtesy of TerraRecon, Inc., San Mateo, CA; with permission.)

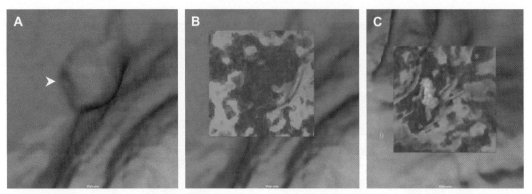

*Fig. 6.* Transparency tool with stool tagging. (*A*) A 7-mm polyp is seen (*arrowhead*). (*B* and *C*) The transparency tool uses a color map to show the density of various pixels. Red represents the soft tissue polyp. Elsewhere in the colon, stool tagged with barium is depicted using this color map as white with a red border. The colon wall is green. (*Courtesy of* Viatronix, Inc., Stony Brook, NY; with permission.)

## Novel views

Conventional endoluminal 3D display modes have some drawbacks. Up to 20% of the colonic mucosa is not examined by a unidirectional fly-through [16]. These hidden zones are located mainly behind semicircular folds that become prominent when there is suboptimal colonic distention and in patients who have diverticulosis accompanied by myochosis ("muscular hypertrophy"). Therefore to examine the entire colon, a fly-through should be

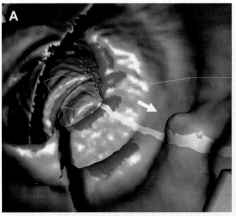

(c) Polyp 2 viewed in the supine scan

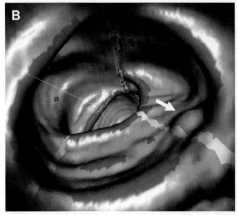

(d) Polyp 2 viewed in the prone scan

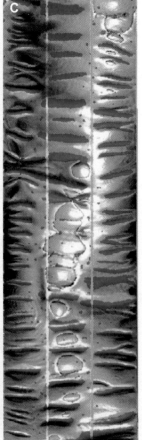

*Fig. 7.* Synchronous navigation system. (*A*) Supine. (*B*) Prone. (*C*) Flattened view. A polyp (*arrow* in *A* and *B*) is seen is the same location on supine and prone views. The position of the virtual camera is controlled based on matching of teniae coli, multiple computer-generated grid lines, and distance from rectum. This system permits a much more accurate and user-friendly comparison of the supine and prone views. The grid lines (blue) and teniae (green and yellow) can be color coded and also displayed in a flattened view (*C*). (*From* Huang A, Roy D, Franaszak M, et al. Teniae coli guided navigation and registration for virtual colonoscopy. In: Silva C, Rushmeier H, Groller E, editors. Proceedings of the IEEE visualization, October 23–28, 2005. Minneapolis (MN): IEEE Press; 2005. p. 279–85; with permission.)

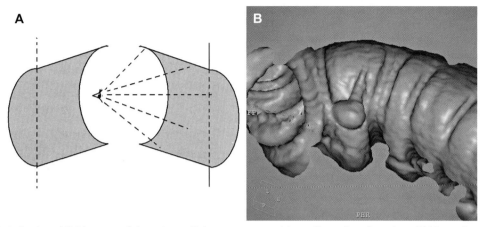

*Fig. 8.* Split view. (*A*) Diagram of the colon split into two cups without flattening the colon. (*B*) View of one half of the split colon. This technique avoids the morphing and distortion associated with flattening. (*Courtesy of Philips Medical Systems, Inc, Bothell, WA; with permission.*)

performed in both antegrade and retrograde directions for both supine and prone positions (a total of four fly-throughs). This process is time consuming and potentially fatiguing.

To overcome these problems, a number of vendors and researchers have developed several novel 3D display methods [2–7]. One method is to "cut the colon open" or "lay it flat" for viewing a part of or the entire colon. To work well, these methods require a well-distended colon. Some programs enable a simultaneous visualization of the colon in antegrade and retrograde directions and of the entire colonic wall with depiction of all the hidden zones. This visualization reduces the 3D examination of the colon to one fly-through per acquisition and should result in a more time-efficient examination. Because more data are projected on the screen simultaneously, however, time is still required for

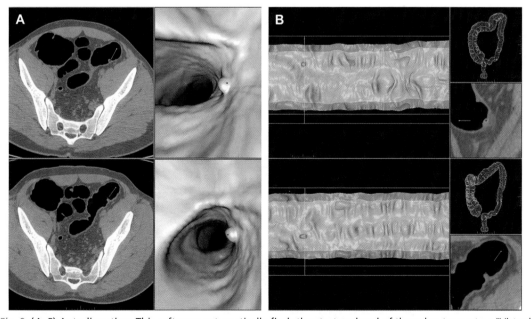

*Fig. 9.* (*A, B*) Autodissection. This software automatically finds the start and end of the colon to create a "Virtual Dissection" view. (*A*) Left panel from a dual monitor showing simultaneous supine and prone axial and 3D endoluminal views. (*B*) Right panel from a dual monitor showing the simultaneous supine and prone virtual dissection views and small thumbnail transparency and orthogonal views. The thumbnail double-contrast barium enema–like transparency views can be enlarged to fill the screen with one mouse click.

the reader to inspect the entire image displayed on the screen, which may be challenging to view for interpretation. Typically any novel view results in some distortion ("morphing") of the colonic structures, making interpretation more difficult. Some vendors have software that can cut the colon open in half without laying it flat to avoid the distortion problem (Fig. 8). In this article the authors discuss and give examples of only a few of these novel views. Because of the large number of vendors offering CTC software, it is not possible to include all of them in this article.

### Virtual pathology/dissection

Various researchers and vendors use different terms to describe a view of the colon as though it were cut open and laid out flat on a table [3,4]. The Virtual Dissection (VD) (GE Healthcare, Inc., Piscataway, New Jersey) program cuts the colon open and displays it either in segments or showing the entire colon in one screen. The user can choose a layout that permits viewing the supine and prone views in VD, 3D endoluminal, and 2D simultaneously with point-to-point correlation between all views (Fig. 9A, B). Simultaneously, a thumbnail 3D transparency view of the colon can be used to assist in assessing colonic anatomy and distention, polyp localization, and comparison of supine and prone positioning. Some investigators advocate using the VD for a fast primary reading [3] and have learned to recognize the reproducible peculiarity of the polyp distortion. Alternately, the VD serves as a fast back-up reading of the entire colon. As with

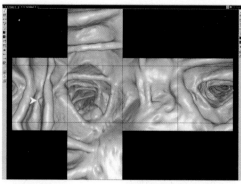

**Fig. 11.** Unfolded Cube View displays the colon forward, backward, and on all four sides. Seamless continuity of the views produces some distortion but shows all surfaces simultaneously. A polyp is seen on a fold (*white arrowhead*). (*Courtesy of* Philips Medical Systems, Inc. Bothell, WA; with permission.)

any similar open view of the colon, VD may help find polyps on either side of a fold.

### Filet view

Although similar to other cut-open views, the filet view creates a movie loop of the cut-open colon displayed for a short segment at a time (see Fig. 4) [5]. This view forces the reader to concentrate on reading one area at a time for a primary reading, but it can be used to correlate with 2D or endoluminal 3D views. There is an interesting and desirable distortion of the fold as it moves across the center of screen, in which the right aspect of the fold is seen a bit better as it approaches the center of the

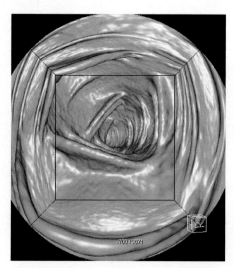

**Fig. 10.** Panoramic view showing an extended view of the colon at the periphery of the image enabling a look at the posterior side of the semicircular folds. There is more distortion at the periphery of the field of view however.

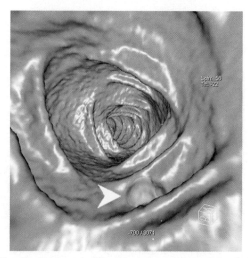

**Fig. 12.** Panoramic 3D with color coding of stool. A computer-aided detection program has found a raised lesion and correctly color coded it as stool (*white arrow*).

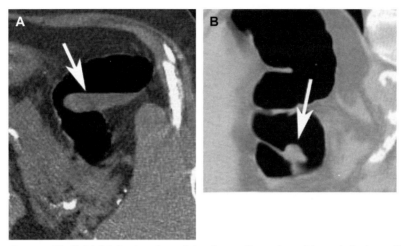

*Fig. 13.* Polyp submerged in fluid. (*A*) Supine view of the descending colon with a relatively small fluid level (*arrow*) that obscures a polyp. (*B*) The prone view reveals the polyp (*arrow*). The comparison of these views emphasizes the need to examine all views meticulously and to perform additional decubitus views when excessive fluid is present.

screen and the left aspect is seen a bit better as the fold passes the center of the screen.

### Panoramic views

Another novel approach to 3D visualization proposes a panoramic endoluminal view. This 3D view enlarges the regular endoluminal view at its margins. This view also shows the colon in both the antegrade and retrograde direction in the same window. The view can be compared with looking at the end of a sleeve that is being rolled up (Fig. 10). The inner part represents the antegrade view of the colon, and the part being rolled up enables to the reader to look behind the semicircular folds and represents the retrograde view of the colon. This method requires more attention from the reader because a larger surface of the colonic wall is shown at once.

### Unfolded cube view

To avoid image distortion, the colon is presented as an Unfolded Cube (Philips Medical Systems, Inc. Bothell, Washington) showing the entire colonic wall on six squares (Fig. 11) [6]. Using the central colonic path, a 90° view is obtained in the six directions: anterior and posterior, up- and downside, and right and left side. These six views then are joined to one unfolded cube view. This display results in a simultaneous projection and visualization of the four parts of the colonic wall (up, down,

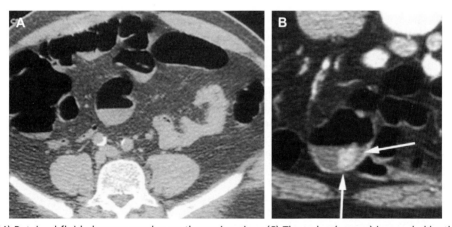

*Fig. 14.* (*A*) Retained fluid obscures a polyp on the supine view. (*B*) The polyp (*arrows*) is revealed by the use of intravenous contrast injection. The use of intravenous contrast agent is an alternate way to help detect polyps in patients who are found to have a large amount of excessive fluid on one view. The decision to administer contrast, with the attendant expense and risk, must be made at the time of the examination.

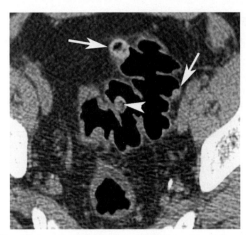

*Fig. 15.* Inverted diverticulum. Displayed best in soft tissue window settings are two diverticula. One is stool filled (*arrow*), and a second is inverted (*arrowhead*). An inverted diverticulum can be diagnosed by tracing pericolonic fat into the center of the apparent intraluminal "lesion."

right, left) and of the colonic lumen in antegrade and retrograde directions. Because a 90° view is used, there is no distortion at the periphery of the image. In a study of 30 patients, Vos and colleagues [6] obtained visualization of 99.5% of the colonic wall with a total evaluation time of 19.5 to 20 minutes, which in this study was significantly shorter than the conventional 3D approach.

### Special considerations for viewing stool tagging

Tagged high-density fluid should be interrogated in wide bone windows (see Fig. 2) to help find submerged polyps [21,22]. This investigation often is done best in a view that is oriented to the plane of the air–fluid level, such as axial or sagittal views. When barium is used to tag solid stool with a minimal or "prepless" CTC [23], the densely tagged areas also should be viewed with wide bone windows to search for a polyp embedded in stool. When a primary 3D reading or a novel view is used, tagged fluid can be subtracted electronically (see Fig. 4), but pieces of tagged stool cannot be subtracted by currently available commercial software. Color mapping using the translucency rendering view can help identify tagged stool directly on 3D views, however (see Fig. 6) [17]. A red color indicates regions with high attenuation. Therefore, a polyp has a red center and shifts to blue over green at its borders. Other software programs can color-code tagged stool on 2D or 3D views (Fig. 12). The reader can differentiate tagged stool, which appears white on the translucency view, if the density of the tagged stool is 200 Hounsfield units or greater.

## Common pitfalls in virtual colonoscopy

There are numerous common and uncommon pitfalls in CTC interpretation, many of which have been discussed in peer-reviewed literature and in texts [24–26]. Often, a problem on 2D can be solved in 3D, or vice versa. For example, distinguishing a polyp from a fold is best done using a 3D view. Recognizing the heterogeneous texture of stool is best achieved using the 2D image while adjusting the window and level in difficult cases. Comparison of supine and prone views is the best approach to show mobility of residual fecal matter, but one must be aware that mobility of the colon itself can lead the reader to mistake a real polyp for stool. Similarly, a pedunculated polyp can move, and a long thin stalk can be overlooked on 2D views. The CTC reader needs to recognize common and uncommon pitfalls such as stool, stool impacted in a diverticulum, fluid obscuring a polyp on one view (Fig. 13) that can be detected only on the contralateral view or by use of intravenous contrast (Fig. 14), unusual but normal folds, flexural pseudotumor, inverted diverticula (Fig. 15), ileocecal valve, surgical anastomosis, and ingested matter.

Flat cancers represent a special pitfall for CTC (Fig. 16). Some so-called "flat lesions" (defined as a lesion whose height is one half its diameter) are easy to see, particularly if the lesion is large and protrudes into the gas-filled lumen. With the definition suggested by the Boston Working Group and others [18,27], however, flat lesions are more aptly defined as pancake like lesions whose height is 3 mm or less. These flat lesions may require an intermediate soft tissue window to make them conspicuous to the reader and may be harder to detect on 3D views [12]. For this reason it is suggested that all CTC cases be viewed in a wide soft tissue window with a specific search performed to find flat lesions.

If artifact is incorrectly identified as a polyp of significant size, the patient may be subjected to unnecessary risks from interventions such as colonoscopy. Conversely, if a true polyp is misinterpreted as stool or artifact, the patient may unknowingly be at significant risk for colorectal cancer.

Most commonly, CTC pitfalls involve retained fluid or stool. Retained fluid has the potential to disguise smaller polyps, decreasing the sensitivity of CTC. For that reason, some suggest using "dry preps" with magnesium citrate. Dry preps, however, tend to leave behind more fecal matter. If there is question about whether the lesion represents retained barium, the examiner should look for a high-attenuating center on 2D views as an aid. Retained stool also often causes difficulty for the reader. Differentiation may be aided by mobility of the lesion in subsequent views, internal

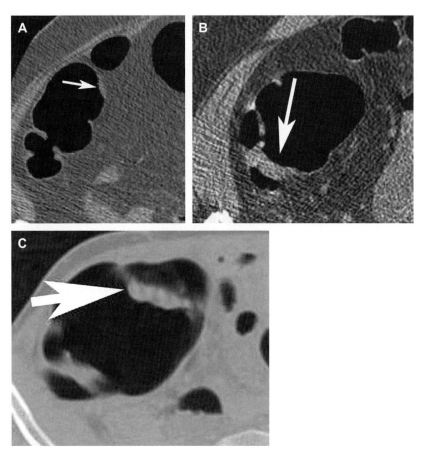

*Fig. 16.* Flat lesions in three different patients. (*A*) A small flat adenoma (*arrow*) seen best on soft tissue windows and confirmed with follow-up CT and endoscopy. (*B*) A larger flat lesion in the ascending colon (*arrow*). (*C*) A flat lesion (*arrow*) was missed on axial images and could be easily confused for ileocecal valve on both axial and 3D views, but on MPR it was conspicuously separate from a normal ileocecal valve. It was proven to be a flat cancer.

heterogeneity, or the presence of barium. Even polyps, however, can trap air against a haustral fold or bowel wall and mimic stool. When distinguishing polyp from stool, it is important to keep bowel motility in mind, because a mobile bowel can leave the impression of lesion mobility. In addition, it may be difficult to differentiate flat lesions from retained stool. With inadequate bowel preparation and significant retained stool, large polyps may be overlooked if there is concomitant poor colonic distention or diverticulosis. If there is any uncertainty about a colonic lesion, colonoscopy should be recommended for further evaluation. Also, tiny foci of relative low density could be present within true polyps (Fig. 17).

Sometimes normal or variant anatomy may cause difficulty during a CTC evaluation. Hemorrhoids may mimic a polyp in the rectum. In this case, there should be correlation with a rectal examination. It also is important to be able to identify a prolapsed appendix in the cecum [28]. Viewing the image in

a soft-tissue window may help with the differentiation. Also in the cecum, it is important to distinguish a prominent ileocecal valve from a mass. In a 3D endoluminal view, the ileocecal valve may appear rounded and elevated. It is important to correlate these findings with 2D images, and the examiner should look carefully for any fat attenuation [29]. Other lesions that may mimic polyps include endometriosis, remnant ovary, colonic lymphocyst, and external compression by the spleen. Sometimes respiratory artifact at the breath-hold interface or motion artifact from the CT table may mimic polyps. In these instances, it is critical to use both 2D MPR and 3D views to aid in correct identification.

With the recent emergence of automated polyp measurements in computer-aided diagnosis, several limitations must be kept in mind. With manual polyp measurements using 2D MPR and 3D views, there is concern about the inter- and intraobserver reliability. Inter- and intraobserver reliability

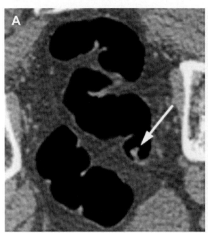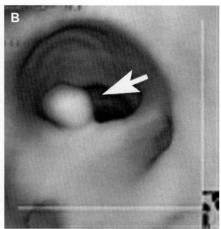

*Fig. 17.* Polyp with atypical density. (*A*) Axial image showed a lesion with focal central low density (*arrow*) suggesting that it might be stool, but the lesion did not move when supine and prone views were compared, and the low density was not distributed diffusely throughout the lesion. (*B*) On endoluminal view the lesion (*arrow*) was smooth surfaced, suggesting a polyp. Endoscopy confirmed a 10-mm adenoma. Only diffuse, mottled low density in a polypoid abnormality reliably indicates stool.

improves significantly with automated measurements, but there is question about the accuracy of these measurements. Some studies indicate that the accuracy of automated measurements is influenced by the size of the polyp, the location, and the morphology. There is some evidence that measurements are more accurate for larger polyps, polyps not located on haustral folds, and pedunculated polyps. Therefore, automated measurements with currently available software may have limited application for flat lesions or lesions on haustral folds. Automated measurements on 3D endoluminal views also may overestimate the lesion and include surrounding haustral fold, ileocecal valve, feces, or fluid. It would be beneficial for radiologists to be able to edit the boundaries on more difficult lesions manually. CAD software also needs to be effective when dealing with electronically subtracted data such as with fecal tagging [30]. Most of the data relating to automated measurements have been reported in cases with adequate colonic distention; however, it would be interesting to see how underdistention affects automated measurements. There is some evidence that increasing colonic distention alters the linear dimensions of small, hyperplastic polyps. As a result, some suggest that automated measurements of volume may allow better surveillance of polyps of intermediate size. Software with this capability has not yet been released or validated, however.

## Summary

Advances and improvements in segmentation, visualization, and reporting software are progressing

rapidly, and products reaching the marketplace often are more advanced than those described in peer-reviewed literature. Advocates of CTC should carefully evaluate these products, many of which are likely to make CTC interpretation more user-friendly. Recognition of pitfalls always will require a skilled interpretation, regardless of the 2D, 3D or novel views used to display the image data.

## Acknowledgments

The authors thank Helen Fenlon, MD, for contributing examples and to the numerous vendors who provided examples of their software.

## Appendix 1

Website addresses of common vendors of CTC software (listed in alphabetical order of company name)

http://www.barco.com/medical/en/solutions/3D_home.asp
http://www.ezem.com/virtual_colon/index.htm
http://www.gehealthcare.com/usen/products.html
http://www.medical.philips.com/us/products/ct/applications/clinical/radiology.html
http://www.rendoscopy.de/
https://www.smed.com/CT/
http://www.terarecon.com/home.html
http://www.vitalimages.com/products/vitrea.aspx
http://www.viatronix.com/

## References

[1] McFarland EG, Pilgram TK, Brink JA, et al. CT colonography: multiobserver diagnostic performance. Radiology 2002;225:380–90.

[2] Paik DS, Beauleau C, Jeffrey RB, et al. Visualization modes for CT colonography using cylindrical and planar map projections. J Comput Assist Tomogr 2000;24:179–88.

[3] Johnson KT, Johnson CD, Fletcher JG, et al. CT colonography using 360-degree virtual dissection: a feasibility study. AJR Am J Roentgenol 2006;186(1):90–5.

[4] Hoppe H, Quattropani C, Spreng A, et al. Virtual colon dissection with CT colonography compared with axial interpretation and conventional colonoscopy: preliminary results. AJR Am J Roentgenol 2004;182:1151–8.

[5] Juchems MS, Fleiter TR, Pauls S, et al. CT colonography: comparison of a colon dissection display versus 3D endoluminal view for the detection of polyps. Eur Radiol 2006;16(1):68–72 [Epub 2005 Jun 14].

[6] Vos FM, van Gelder RE, Serlie IWO, et al. Three-dimensional display modes for conventional 3D virtual colonoscopy versus unfolded cube projection. Radiology 2003;228:878–85.

[7] Geiger B, Chefd'hotel C, Sudarsky S. Panoramic views for virtual endoscopy. Med Image Comput Comput Assist Interv Int Conf Med Image Comput Comput assist Interv 2005;8(Pt 1):662–9.

[8] Dachman AH. Advice for optimizing colonic distension and minimizing risk of perforation during CT colonography. [editorial]. Radiology 2006;239:317–21.

[9] Dachman AH, Kuniyoshi JK, Boyle CM, et al. CT colography with 3D problem solving for detection of colonic polyps. AJR Am J Roentgenol 1998;171:989–95.

[10] Macari M, Milano A, Lavelle M, et al. Comparison of time-efficient CT colonography with two- and three-dimensional colonic evaluation for detecting colorectal polyps. AJR Am J Roentgenol 2000;174:1543–9.

[11] Macari M, Megibow AJ. Pitfalls of using three-dimensional CT colonography with two-dimensional imaging correlation. AJR Am J Roentgenol 2001;176:137–43.

[12] Fidler JL, Johnson CD, MacCarty RL, et al. Detection of flat lesions in the colon with CT colonography. Abdom Imaging 2002;27:292–300.

[13] Laks S, Macari M, Bini EJ. Positional change in colon polyps at CT colonography. Radiology 2004;231:761–6.

[14] Chen JC, Dachman AH. CT colonography: cecal mobility as a potential pitfall. AJR Am J Roentgenol 2006;186:1086–9.

[15] Zalis ME, Perumpillichira JJ, Magee C, et al. Tagging-based, electronically cleansed CT colonography: evaluation of patient comfort and image readability. Radiology 2006;239(1):149–59 [erratum in: Radiology. 2006; 240(1):304].

[16] Pickhardt PJ, Taylor AJ, Gopal DV. Surface visualization at 3D endoluminal CT colonography: degree of coverage and implications for polyp detection. Gastroenterology 2006;130(6):1582–7.

[17] Pickhardt PJ. Translucency rendering in 3D endoluminal CT colonography: a useful tool for increasing polyp specificity and decreasing interpretation time. AJR Am J Roentgenol 2004; 183:429–36.

[18] Zalis ME, Barish MA, Choi JR, et al. CT colonography reporting and data system: a consensus proposal. Radiology 2005;236:3–9.

[19] Pickhardt PJ, Lehman VT, Winter TC, et al. Polyp volume versus linear size measurements at CT colonography: implications for noninvasive surveillance of unresected colorectal lesions. AJR Am J Roentgenol 2006;186(6):1605–10.

[20] Huang A, Summers RM, Roy D. Synchronous navigation for CT colonography. In: Manduca A, Amini AA, editors. Medical imaging 2006: physiology, function, and structure from medical images Proceedings of the SILE; 2006. Abstract 614315.

[21] Lefere PA, Gryspeerdt SS, Dewyspelaere J, et al. Dietary fecal tagging as a cleansing method before CT colonography: initial results polyp detection and patient acceptance. Radiology 2002;224:393–403.

[22] Dachman AH, Dawson DO, Lefere P, et al. Comparison of routine and unprepped CT colonography augmented by low fiber diet and stool tagging: a pilot study. Abdom Imaging 2006 Sep 13; [Epub ahead of print].

[23] Iannaccone R, Laghi A, Catalano C, et al. CTC without cathartic preparation for the detection of colorectal polyps. Gastroenterology 2004;27:1300–11.

[24] Taylor SA, Halligan S, Bartram CI. CT colonography: methods, pathology and pitfalls. Clin Radiol 2003;58:179–90.

[25] Dachman AH, editor. Atlas of virtual colonoscopy. New York: Springer-Verlag, Inc.; 2003.

[26] Gryspeerdt S, Lefere P. How to avoid pitfalls in imaging: causes and solutions to overcome false negatives and false positives. In: Lefere P, Gryspeerdt S, editors. Medical radiology—diagnostic imaging. Virtual colonoscopy: a practical guide. Berlin: Springer-Verlag; 2006. p. 87–116.

[27] Dachman AH, Zalis ME. Quality and consistency in CT colonography and research reporting. Radiology 2004;230:319–23.

[28] Gollub MJ. Inverted appendiceal orifice masquerading as a cecal polyp on virtual colonoscopy. Gastrointest Endosc 2006;63(2):358.

[29] Yitta S, Tatineny KC, Cipriani NA, et al. Characterization of normal ileocecal valve density on CT colonography. J Comput Assist Tomogr 2006;30(1):58–61.

[30] Yoshida H, Dachman AH. Computer-aided diagnosis for CT colonography. Seminars in Ultrasound CT MR 2004;25:419–31.

RADIOLOGIC
CLINICS
OF NORTH AMERICA

Radiol Clin N Am 45 (2007) 361–375

ELSEVIER
SAUNDERS

# CT Colonography (Virtual Colonoscopy): A Practical Approach for Population Screening

Perry J. Pickhardt, MD*, David H. Kim, MD

- Program set-up
  *Third-party coverage*
  *Support and personnel*
  *Clinical colleagues*
- CT colonography technique
  *Colonic preparation*
  *Colonic distention*
  *Multidetector protocol*

- CT colonography interpretation
  *Biphasic polyp detection*
  *Diagnostic algorithm*
  *Diagnostic pitfalls*
- Summary
- References

CT colonography (CTC), also referred to as "virtual colonoscopy," is ideally suited for population screening of asymptomatic adults. Colorectal cancer, although largely preventable or at least curable if detected early, remains a major killer because of poor compliance with existing screening strategies. At the University of Wisconsin Hospital and Clinics (UWHC), the use of a proven method for CTC has paved the way for local third-party reimbursement for screening, which was initiated in April 2004 [1,2]. This article describes the procedural details of the authors' current approach to CTC screening, which has evolved steadily and matured over time. The discussion focuses primarily on program set-up, CTC study technique, and study interpretation. For the interested reader, a somewhat more detailed account of the authors' specific CTC technique and interpretation can be found elsewhere [3]. It is not the authors' intention to provide an exhaustive review of the CTC literature or to compare all the different CTC techniques currently in use. Instead, they hope to provide a practical approach to CTC screening that conveys some of the lessons that they have learned during the development of their own clinical program. Many of the hurdles that they have encountered along the way can be lessened or removed altogether for those that wish to follow on the path of CTC screening.

## Program set-up

Institution of any new clinical program typically entails a series of both predictable and unforeseen challenges and obstacles. Currently, the general lack of reimbursement for CTC screening results in a "catch-22" situation: clinical experience is needed to demonstrate local efficacy of CTC screening, but it is difficult to generate sufficient volume without third-party coverage. This section also discusses briefly a host of other administrative set-up issues that should be considered.

Department of Radiology, University of Wisconsin Medical School, E3/311 Clinical Science Center, 600 Highland Ave., Madison, WI 53792-3252, USA
* Corresponding author.
*E-mail address:* pj.pickhardt@hosp.wisc.edu (P.J. Pickhardt).

doi:10.1016/j.rcl.2007.03.011

## Third-party coverage

When the authors were first setting up their program at UWHC in 2004, the outlook for CTC screening reimbursement at the national level was not favorable. Therefore, the authors instead undertook a "grass roots" approach to try to convince third-party payers at the local level. Dane County, Wisconsin, is fairly well penetrated by managed care organizations (MCOs) that have some ability to make local coverage decisions. At a February 2004 technology assessment meeting at UWHC that included the medical directors of all the major MCOs, the authors argued the case for third-party coverage of screening CTC examinations performed at UWHC [4]. In general, the need for additional effective and available screening options for the prevention and detection of colorectal cancer was clear. Specifically, the authors were able to ensure these directors that a proven method for CTC screening would be used, pointing to the Department of Defense multicenter clinical trial that had just been completed in March 2003 and published in the *New England Journal of Medicine* in December 2003 [1]. Support from some of the authors' gastroenterology colleagues provided additional credibility. Shortly after this meeting, the MCOs decided to approve reimbursement for this specific method of CTC, including both screening and diagnostic examinations [4]. Although it was recognized that coverage of an additional option for screening probably would lead to greater resource use, the MCOs determined that this coverage is a judicious use of premium dollars and probably is cost effective in the long run. The authors formally began reimbursed CTC screening at UWHC in April 2004. To their knowledge, no other program to date has achieved similar third-party coverage for screening CTC. More recently, they also have been successful in significantly broadening Medicare coverage for diagnostic CTC through a major overhaul of an initially restrictive local coverage determination for diagnostic CTC. Of course, any Medicare decision to cover screening CTC would require national action.

The current prospects for national or regional coverage of CTC screening by third-party payers seem to hinge on the support from a variety of professional societies, technology assessment groups, task forces, and so on. The American Cancer Society is in the process of reviewing its guidelines for recommended colorectal screening tests, which currently include the barium enema but not CTC. A number of other groups and organizations probably will wait until the ongoing American College of Radiology Imaging Network (ACRIN) CTC trial (Study 6664) ends, although final results may not be available until late 2007. If the ultimate results of the ACRIN trial are favorable, additional CTC software systems will be validated for screening, and more widespread third-party reimbursement probably will follow quickly. Even if the ACRIN results are disappointing, however, they do not detract from the CTC methods that already have been validated for screening. Perhaps this latter scenario will pave the way for a consensus on successful CTC screening approaches, leaving behind those that have failed repeatedly. At the very least, one feasible approach might be to create "centers of excellence," like UWHC, that use only validated screening CTC techniques. In actuality, such centers could be in operation already, with third-party coverage, if a local approach, similar to that the authors instituted, were applied.

## Support and personnel

The technical requirements for setting up a CTC program are not demanding, because nearly all radiology practices have the key equipment already in place (ie, a multidetector CT scanner). The CTC software and an automated carbon dioxide delivery device represent relatively minor capital investments (although the choice of specific software is, of course, critical). Beyond equipment needs, however, it is essential not to overlook the importance of dedicated personnel. A motivated clinical program coordinator, preferably with some nursing or other clinical background, is particularly helpful for handling the unforeseen administrative difficulties associated with setting up a new program [4]. Given that an estimated 40 million adults over 50 years of age have not been screened properly, the potential for unprecedented new growth that CTC screening can bring to a practice is clear, as the authors have already experienced. As such, the investment in a new coordinator position can be justified easily. As discussed later, it also is important for the technical quality of the CTC studies to obtain the trust and support from the CT technologists who will be involved. Other potential administrative challenges worth considering include patient scheduling and follow-up, database management, prep kit assembly and distribution, program marketing and Website design, and colonoscopy referral.

## Clinical colleagues

Because many discussions surrounding the appropriate role of CTC in screening seem to involve gastroenterology colleagues, it is easy to forget that they do not represent the actual patient-referral base. Rather, the gatekeepers who decide which test to order for their patients are the primary care providers, such as general practitioners and internists. Therefore, although approval from gastroenterology can provide some needed credibility early on, it is not absolutely essential as long as the referring physicians understand the value and advantages of CTC screening. Education through grand rounds presentations and other forms of communication can help build support for a fledgling CTC screening program. Unlike mammography screening, the authors have chosen to require physician referral for CTC screening, so as not to disengage or alienate them from the process. This helps foster a more collegial referral base and provides an important link when additional work up is required for a potentially significant extracolonic finding identified on CTC.

With regards to colorectal screening, close cooperation between radiology and gastroenterology can be mutually beneficial. With both groups working together, patients can benefit by undergoing the most appropriate study. Most importantly, overall compliance with screening can be increased by allowing patients a choice between optical and virtual options for total colonic examination. For example, just 1 year after the introduction of the CTC program, the total number of patients being screened at UWHC more than doubled [2]. In addition, patient referral for diagnostic studies is a two-way street, because optical colonoscopy is needed for removal of significant lesions found at CTC, and CTC is needed for incomplete optical colonoscopy or for further evaluation of certain submucosal masses. At UWHC, the option for same-day optical colonoscopy is offered for significant lesions detected at CTC, a convenience highly valued by the authors' patients because it ensures complete care with a single bowel preparation. Providing the gastroenterologist with detailed CTC images depicting polyp location and appearance (Fig. 1) can streamline and even improve overall patient care, because some difficult lesions probably would be missed at colonoscopy if not for the advance knowledge of their presence given by CTC.

## CT colonography technique

The general idea behind CTC is fairly straightforward. When multidetector CT (MDCT) is used to image a properly prepared and distended colon, clinically relevant polyps can be readily detected with dedicated CTC software [5]. If all facets of CTC examination are addressed adequately, effective evaluation is relatively easy. Any weak link, however, can lead to poor results. For example, even the best CTC software system will fail if there is inadequate colonic preparation or distention. Likewise, optimal preparation and distention cannot compensate for an inadequate software system or an ineffective interpretive approach. This section briefly reviews the authors' methods for bowel preparation, colonic distention, and MDCT scanning.

### Colonic preparation

Robust preparation is critical for accurate polyp detection at CTC and requires both cleansing and tagging. The authors' current low-volume CTC preparation has proven successful and combines three basic components: (1) a laxative for catharsis, (2) 250 mL dilute 2% barium for tagging of any solid residual stool, and (3) 60 mL water-soluble iodinated contrast (diatrizoate) for opacification of luminal fluid [3]. This preparation has been greatly simplified from the authors' multicenter trial, and they have yet to encounter any significant preparation-related complications. In addition to the preparation itself, the patient maintains a clear liquid diet the day before the examination. The specific laxative used depends on the health status of the individual. The authors provide referring physicians with their guidelines and have them choose the most appropriate cathartic agent for their patients.

The authors' standard laxative is sodium phosphate, which is employed in more than 85% of cases and is well tolerated in screening adults without known or suspected renal or cardiac insufficiency. In addition, they generally avoid sodium phosphate in elderly patients who have hypertension, particularly those taking angiotensin-converting enzyme inhibitors [6]. Although they never experienced a problem using two 45-mL doses of sodium phosphate spaced 3 hours apart during the screening trial, they since have shown that a single dose is equally effective [7], which brings their preparation into compliance with Food and Drug Administration (FDA) regulations. If further purgation is needed, patients now are encouraged to take a bottle of magnesium citrate in lieu of a second dose of sodium phosphate. From a practical standpoint, most patients find it easier to drink the undiluted sodium phosphate rapidly, followed immediately by a clear liquid chaser, such as a carbonated beverage. Alternatively, the solution can be diluted into an 8-oz glass of clear juice or soda.

For nearly all patients in whom sodium phosphate is best avoided, magnesium citrate represents an acceptable substitute and is given as a 296-mL bottle. Because the authors find it somewhat less effective than sodium phosphate, a second bottle is taken long with the 2% barium. For severely compromised patients who cannot tolerate even moderate fluid or electrolyte shifts, the authors resort to polyethylene glycol, which is given as a 4-L solution. Although the safety profile of polyethylene glycol is most favorable for such tenuous patients,

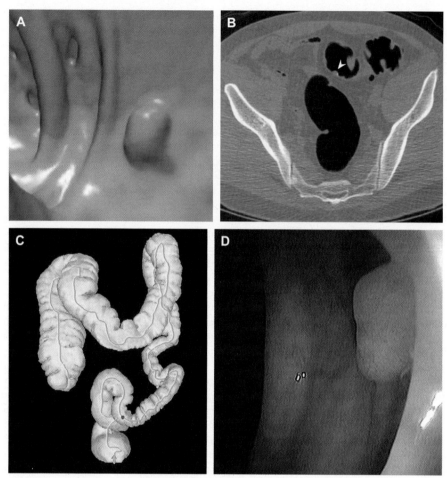

*Fig. 1.* Colonic polyp detected at CTC screening. (*A*) 3D endoluminal CTC image shows a 9-mm polyp in the sigmoid colon. Note the diverticula in the background. (*B*) 2D transverse CTC image confirms that the polyp (*arrowhead*) is composed of soft tissue density. Note how the thickened sigmoid folds have a polypoid appearance, which greatly complicates the 2D search pattern but does not interfere with confirmation of a 3D finding. (*C*) 3D colonic map shows the precise location of the polyp (*red dot*). This information, along with 3D polyp images in panel A and 2D polyp images in panel B, is provided to the gastroenterologist before optical colonoscopy to facilitate detection. The green line indicates the automated centerline for endoluminal navigation. (*D*) Digital photograph from optical colonoscopy performed the same day as CTC shows the corresponding polyp, which proved to be hyperplastic. Because the polyp was in the 6- to 9-mm range, the patient also had the option for CTC surveillance according to the UWHC protocol.

this preparation is associated with the poorest compliance because of its consistency and large volume. Fortunately, this preparation is rarely necessary for screening CTC, accounting for less than 1% of the authors' cases.

Regardless of the laxative used, the dual oral contrast regimen is held constant. The authors believe that the complementary actions of the dilute barium and diatrizoate provide optimal CTC preparation [8]. As with the sodium phosphate, the total volume of each oral contrast agent has been cut in half and reduced to a single dose, without any discernible detriment to the fidelity of the preparation. The basic rationale behind the specific order of the three preparation components is that the laxative provides catharsis for the bulk removal of fecal material, the barium tags any residual solid stool that remains, and the diatrizoate serves the dual purpose of uniform fluid tagging and secondary catharsis (Fig. 2) [8,9]. The authors strongly prefer dilute 2% CT barium over 30% to 40% barium, which is unnecessarily dense, less well tolerated, and may even cause problems for same-day colonoscopy. In the authors' experience, the 2% barium has never caused a significant problem in the more than 1500 same-day colonoscopy studies performed following CTC. They suspect that the diatrizoate represents their true "secret to success." It uniformly opacifies

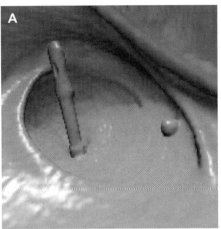 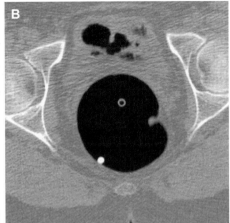

*Fig. 2.* Adherent tagged stool simulating a polyp on 3D. (*A*) Prone 3D endoluminal CTC image shows a small polypoid lesion within the rectum. Note the small caliber rectal catheter. (*B*) Corresponding prone 2D transverse CTC image shows that the lesion represents tagged adherent stool.

the residual luminal fluid and provides secondary catharsis; it also has a "slippery" consistency that seems to decrease greatly the amount of adherent solid debris. The last feature is key, because adherent stool can be a major source of false positives, but mobile stool in the fluid pool causes no difficulty, unless electronic fluid subtraction is performed (a technique the authors no longer use). In the authors' limited experience with nonionic iodinated contrast (eg, iohexol), they believe that the increase in adherent residual stool unfortunately outweighs the more palatable taste.

The use of dual oral contrast tagging improves the accuracy of CTC in several ways: it increases specificity by both tagging residual stool (barium effect) and decreasing the amount of adherent stool (diatrizoate effect), and it increases sensitivity by allowing polyp detection in opacified fluid (diatrizoate effect). Given the improved performance characteristics seen with the use of oral contrast tagging, it should be considered standard CTC technique and should be used whenever possible. In the authors' experience with same-day CTC following incomplete optical colonoscopy, the lack of contrast tagging has resulted in a number of false positives that almost certainly would have been eliminated with dedicated CTC preparation. Attempts at secondary oral contrast administration in this setting also have been disappointing, forcing the authors to reconsider same-day CTC in some cases. With regard to computer-aided detection, most algorithms to date have been developed and tested on cases without tagging. To move forward successfully, the authors believe that computer-aided detection systems will need to address this issue and demonstrate acceptable performance for tagged cases [10,11].

## Colonic distention

Adequate luminal distension of the colon, like proper bowel preparation, is a critical component of technical success. Adequate distention does not necessarily indicate maximal distention, because patient comfort and safety must be taken into account if CTC is to be widely embraced. The authors' distention protocol has continued to evolve and improve, resulting in inadequate segmental distention in less than 1% of all patients. The use of large, rigid retention balloon catheters designed for the barium enema is rarely indicated for CTC screening. In the authors' experience, the small-caliber, flexible catheters with low-pressure retention cuffs specifically designed for CTC work very well.

For a number of reasons, automated $CO_2$ delivery represents the author's front-line distention technique, with room air insufflation serving as a seldom-used back up. Of note, nearly all reported perforations at CTC have involved the use of manual staff-controlled room air insufflation, whereas the risk of perforation with automated or patient-controlled distention methods probably approaches zero for screening CTC [12]. In both degree of distention and postprocedural discomfort, automated $CO_2$ seems superior to manual room air technique [13]. One additional factor that receives little attention is nonetheless very important: staff preference. The authors' CT technologists strongly prefer the automated $CO_2$ technique to room air insufflation. Significant time and energy may be required to coach individual patients to self-insufflate with room air adequately, whereas automated $CO_2$ requires little explanation, and end-point determination is more straightforward. From the radiologist's perspective, the decreased operator dependence with the automated $CO_2$ technique results in less variability between studies.

The authors believe that spasmolytics generally are unnecessary and are best avoided for CTC screening [13]. Previous studies evaluating the efficacy of spasmolytics have found mixed but largely negative results. Furthermore, the needle administration of a drug adds to invasiveness and patient discomfort, creates an opportunity for possible new side effects, increases the duration of the examination, and increases overall costs. Finally, with the authors' current distention protocol, nondiagnostic segmental distention is so rare that the potential role for spasmolytics is diminished greatly from the start. Even if there were a mild net benefit with hyoscine butylbromide compared with glucagon, this agent is not currently available in the United States.

Over time, the authors have refined their protocol for colonic distention. To maintain efficiency, they have trained their CT technologists to obtain the entire CTC examination, including placement of the rectal catheter. The radiologist is needed only for difficult or unusual situations, thus allowing more time for study interpretation. Immediately before the examination begins, the patient is encouraged to use the bathroom, and the technologist inquires about the fidelity of the preparation. After rectal catheter placement, the patient remains in the left lateral decubitus position for the initial 1 to 1.5 L $CO_2$ delivered by the automated device (PROTOCO$_2$L, E-Z-EM Inc, Westbury, NY). To reduce transient discomfort related to rectal spasm, the authors initially set the equilibrium pressure at about 20 mm Hg. The patient then is placed in the right lateral decubitus position until about 2.5 L has been delivered in total, followed by supine positioning until a steady-state equilibrium has been reached, at which time scanning commences. The positional change generally prevents underdistention related to $CO_2$ blockage from a fluid channel. The volume of $CO_2$ dispensed can vary widely because of actual differences in colonic volume and because of variable degrees of reflux through the ileocecal valve, loss around the catheter, and continuous colonic resorption. Therefore, the total volume reading has relatively little meaning and can range from 3 L to more than 10 L in some cases. As a practical point, any $CO_2$ lost from the large intestine must be replaced actively during scanning. The authors perform the supine and prone scans at end expiration to raise the diaphragm and allow more room for the splenic flexure and transverse colon.

Although the CT scout image provides a general indication of overall colonic distention, the authors have found that it is unreliable for assessing distention of the sigmoid and descending colon (Fig. 3) [14]. Consequently, they have trained their CT technologists to recognize inadequate distention immediately on review of the two-dimensional (2D) transverse images during the examination. If focal collapse persists at the same point on both supine and prone scans, a third set of images is obtained in the right lateral decubitus position. These steps ensure adequate distention of the left colon, resulting in nondiagnostic segmental evaluation in less than 1% of cases. In these unusual cases, which almost always are caused by severe diverticular disease, the authors usually offer same-day unsedated flexible sigmoidoscopy (see Fig. 3). In rare instances, manual room air insufflation may help maintain adequate distention when $CO_2$ has failed.

## Multidetector protocol

Unlike temporally demanding protocols like CT angiography, CTC is a very forgiving examination with regard to scanner requirements, for several reasons: (1) screening CTC is a noncontrast study; (2) the gas-filled large intestine is a relatively static structure; and (3) the target lesion is relatively large. Therefore, neither submillimeter collimation nor 64-channel scanners are necessary. On the contrary, the increased dose required for submillimeter collimation probably outweighs any theoretical benefit for polyp detection. In fact, although the authors prefer an 8-channel or 16-channel MDCT scanner with 1.25 collimation, most CTC studies from their screening trial were performed on 4-channel scanners using a $4 \times 2.5$-mm detector configuration [1].

The authors' current CTC protocol remains fairly straightforward. They believe that the well-established practice of obtaining both supine and prone scans should remain, given the invaluable complementary data provided and the ability to confirm suspected lesions detected on one view. Typical 16-channel MDCT scanning factors include a 0.5-second rotation time, 1.25-mm collimation, 1.375:1 pitch, 1.0-mm reconstruction interval, and 120 kV$_p$. Given the nature of the soft tissue–air interface for polyp detection at CTC, it is widely recognized that the radiation dose can be lowered significantly from the usual diagnostic levels. To optimize the delivered dose, the authors prefer to use a tube-current modulation system (Smart mA, GE Medical Systems, Milwaukee, Wisconsin) and set the noise index to its current maximum level of 50, which has yielded significant dose reduction and uniformly diagnostic examinations. For MDCT scanners that are not equipped with a tube-current modulation system, the authors generally employ a technique in the range of 35 to 75 mAs (effective), except for individualized increases in morbidly obese patients. Although further dose

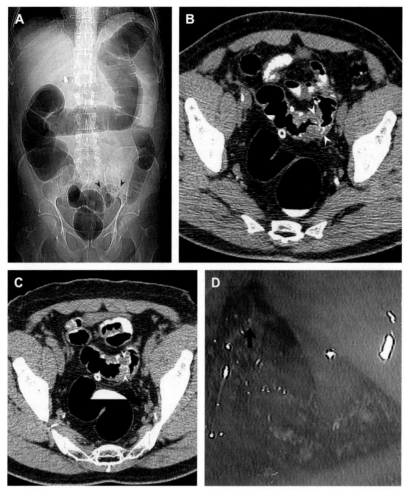

*Fig. 3.* Diverticular stricture of the sigmoid colon. (*A*) Supine CT scout radiograph from screening CTC shows a narrowed luminal caliber to the sigmoid colon (*arrowheads*) related to diverticular disease but no apparent areas of frank collapse or nondistention. The prone scout had a similar appearance (not shown). (*B* and *C*) 2D transverse CTC images with (*B*) supine and (*C*) prone positioning show extensive sigmoid diverticular disease. Importantly, wall thickening with focal luminal nondistention is seen at the same point on both views (*arrowheads*). This appearance remained unchanged on right lateral decubitus positioning (not shown). The patient was offered same-day unsedated flexible sigmoidoscopy for further evaluation of this area. Nondiagnostic segmental evaluation such as this is rarely seen with the authors' current distention protocol, occurring in less than 1% of cases. (*D*) Digital photograph from flexible sigmoidoscopy confirms fixed narrowing from benign diverticular disease (*arrow*). Mild erythema is present from superimposed inflammation.

reduction is obviously a desirable goal for screening evaluation of asymptomatic adults, it is reassuring to note that the very small theoretical risk of low-dose radiation exposure is clearly outweighed by the actual risk of not being screened for colorectal cancer [15,16].

The thin-section source images are sent to the CTC workstation for advanced modeling and interpretation and to the picture archiving and communications system for storage. In addition to the source data, the authors automatically perform a second reconstruction of the supine dataset into a separate series of contiguous 5-mm images [17].

This additional series facilitates review of extracolonic structures by providing fewer images with less image noise. Because of the high diagnostic accuracy of CTC when oral contrast tagging and three-dimensional (3D) polyp detection are employed [1,2], the use of intravenous contrast is not indicated for screening. Without a clear benefit over the authors' noncontrast protocol, the disadvantages of introducing intravenous contrast for CTC screening, such as increased time, costs, invasiveness, and risks, do not warrant its routine use at this time. As an aside, the authors do use an intravenous contrast CTC protocol in the setting of incomplete colonoscopy from an occlusive carcinoma and occasionally for suspected submucosal lesions. In brief, this protocol entails obtaining a low-dose prone scan first, followed by a postcontrast supine scan with standard diagnostic technique.

## CT colonography interpretation

This section describes the authors' interpretive approach and their diagnostic algorithm and reviews a number of common diagnostic pitfalls that should be recognized. Discussion of promising research tools not yet in use for clinical screening, such as computer-aided detection and nonstandard 3D displays (eg, virtual dissection view) are beyond the scope of this practical overview.

### *Biphasic polyp detection*

Redundancy is the key to accurate polyp detection with CTC. The more chances one has to detect a lesion without too much mental strain or intensity of effort, the less likely it is that a significant polyp will be missed. It is critical to understand that the "standard" interpretive approach of "primary 2D with 3D problem solving" is inadequate for low-prevalence CTC screening, primarily because it fails to incorporate the benefit of primary 3D detection. The authors' biphasic interpretive approach emphasizes 3D detection but also retains the complementary value of 2D detection. The existing evidence is clear: of the five large CTC trials to date evaluating low-prevalence cohorts, the three that used a primary 2D approach faired poorly [18–20], whereas the performance in the two trials that used a biphasic

approach was comparable to optical colonoscopy [1,21]. The general concept behind the authors' interpretive approach is that the more sensitive but less specific 3D endoluminal display is best for initial polyp detection, whereas the more specific but less sensitive 2D display is used for confirmation of suspected lesions and for secondary polyp detection. Although 2D is excellent for confirming the soft tissue nature of polyps, it is a rather ineffective and tedious method for detecting them initially, largely because of their poor conspicuity amongst the colonic folds (see Fig. 1). Primary 2D evaluation, however, is particularly helpful for annular lesions, fluid-filled areas (assuming oral contrast tagging has been applied), and segments with partial or total luminal collapse.

Although the published data strongly support the importance of 3D polyp detection, several conditions existing during the early development of CTC may help explain why some still regard primary 2D as the front-line detection method. First, 2D multiplanar reformatted (MPR) displays were already fully mature at this time. Second, radiologists had already gained a comfort level with 2D. Third, a time-efficient 3D endoluminal evaluation was not yet feasible [5]. Consequently, nearly all CTC systems were based initially on the primary 2D paradigm [22]. Some studies intended to compare 2D and 3D detection unfortunately have used CTC systems with either poor or inefficient 3D capabilities. Long interpretation times for 3D endoluminal evaluation are reported by some but these times are highly system dependent and continue to decline rapidly. Furthermore, although primary 2D detection typically can perform well in

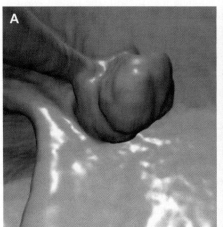
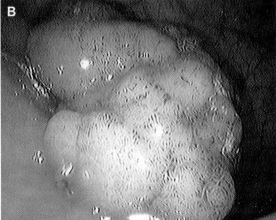

*Fig. 4.* Advanced neoplasm detected at CTC screening. (*A*) 3D endoluminal CTC image shows a 3.5-cm lobulated soft tissue mass, which (*B*) proved to be a large tubulovillous adenoma after polypectomy at same-day optical colonoscopy.

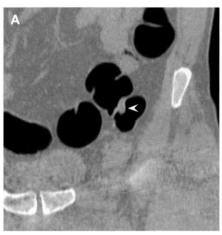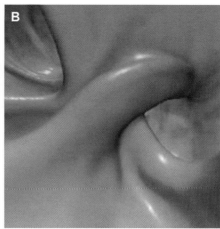

Fig. 5. Prominent fold simulating a polyp on 2D. (A) 2D coronal CTC image shows a focal polypoid appearance (arrowhead) to the colonic folds. (B) On the 3D view, this was found to represent slight torsion of normal colonic folds at a flexure point. Thickened or complex folds create an unnecessarily difficult environment for primary 2D polyp detection.

small, polyp-rich cohorts, it is incorrect to extrapolate such results to the screening setting where finding significant polyps is more akin to finding a needle in a haystack.

The authors initially started out as primary 2D readers, but it became clear over time that many lesions either missed or barely detected on 2D evaluation were obvious on 3D. Because self-discovery is more convincing than force-fed dogma, and because 2D detection remains an important skill, the authors have all trainees in their CTC program begin with primary 2D evaluation until they have gained significant experience. In the authors' experience, the initial learning curve for 3D detection is much easier, and a sustained level of high performance is easier to achieve [3]. Because the polyp search pattern with 3D is so much more relaxed, and because polyps are so much more conspicuous, reader fatigue is much less an issue than with 2D. (video clips) Overall, the authors believe that the reliance on 2D (or reluctance to switch to 3D) for polyp detection is beginning to change, particularly as other CTC software systems continue to improve their 3D capabilities.

"Access video in online version of article at http://www.radiologic.theclinics.com."

At present, the authors use the V3D Colon system (Viatronix Inc., Stony Brook, New York) for CTC interpretation. To their knowledge, this is currently the only CTC system that is FDA-approved for screening, because it has already been proven effective in this setting [1,4]. Software improvements since the time of the authors' screening trial have resulted in ever-faster and more accurate CTC interpretation [2,23]. With the authors' biphasic approach, the reader uses both 3D and 2D polyp detection modes. Almost all significant polyps, however, can be detected readily on the 3D endoluminal, rendering 2D detection supplementary and clearly secondary. Primary 3D review entails bidirectional automated fly-through of the supine and prone models with manual navigation as needed for further inspection of suspicious areas (video clips). Increasing the field-of-view angle to 120 degrees may allow for just a single fly-through on both supine and prone views. A major drawback with the 3D endoluminal display on most other CTC systems is the lack of unrestricted manual navigation. Complete 3D coverage is assured by the system, which continually tracks and updates the fraction of endoluminal surface covered [24]. Rapid interrogation of polypoid lesions detected on 3D can be accomplished by the usual 2D MPR correlation or with 3D translucency rendering that provides information on the internal density of a lesion [25]. When used properly, the translucency-rendering tool can decrease interpretation time by reducing the need for 2D confirmation of false positives, such as tagged stool. For most CTC screening cases, the entire study can be read in 10 minutes or less [23]. Although the Viatronix V3D system allows electronic cleansing of the opacified residual luminal fluid [8,26], the authors have kept this function disabled at UWHC because they believe the artifacts that are introduced currently outweigh the potential benefits [3,5,23].

"Access video in online version of article at http://www.radiologic.theclinics.com."

### Diagnostic algorithm

For patients undergoing colorectal screening with CTC, the largest detected lesion primarily determines the next appropriate step. The authors' diagnostic algorithm is based on polyp-size categories and is similar to the one proposed by the Working Group on Virtual Colonoscopy [27]. Adoption of reasonable polyp-size thresholds is a critical requirement for the ultimate success of CTC screening [28]. There is general agreement that immediate optical colonoscopy for polypectomy is generally warranted for all large polyps (≥ 10 mm) detected at CTC screening. In the authors' experience at UWHC, a large polyp or mass is seen in approximately 1 of every 20 average-risk adults screened (Fig. 4) [29]. Because most of these lesions turn out to be advanced adenomas that represent the target for cancer prevention, the risks of undergoing polypectomy probably are outweighed by the malignant potential of these larger lesions. A screening CTC study is considered positive

when any lesion 6 mm or larger is detected, representing about 12% of asymptomatic adults, in the authors' experience. Although all patients who have medium-sized lesions (6–9 mm) are offered same-day colonoscopy, subcentimeter polyps almost never are malignant and only rarely are histologically advanced [30]. In fact, it remains unclear whether the inherent neoplastic risk of a medium-sized polyp detected at CTC outweighs the procedural risks associated with colonoscopic polypectomy [3,28]. Therefore, under an internal review board–approved protocol, the authors also offer patients the option for short-term CTC surveillance, based on the notion that the majority of lesions should remain stable or regress over time.

Of note, precise linear measurement of polyps is not as straightforward as might seem. The 2D measurement, which always should be optimized

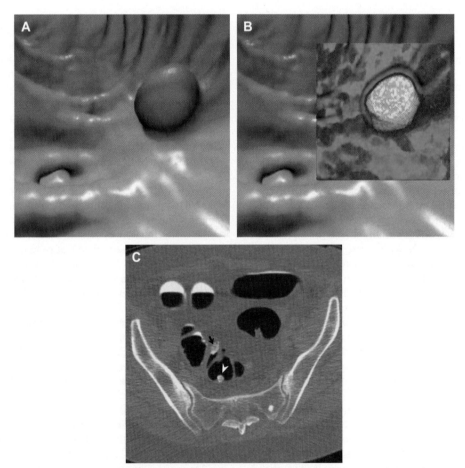

*Fig. 6.* Impacted and inverted diverticulum simulating a polyp on 3D. (*A and B*) Prone 3D endoluminal CTC images (*A*) without and (*B*) with translucency rendering show a polypoid lesion adjacent to a diverticulum. The central white color signature on translucency rendering suggests high internal density and not soft tissue composition. (*C*) Corresponding prone 2D transverse CTC image shows an impacted diverticulum (*arrowhead*) filled with dense stool along the nondependent wall that has prolapsed or inverted into the lumen. Multiple other impacted diverticula were present (*arrow*).

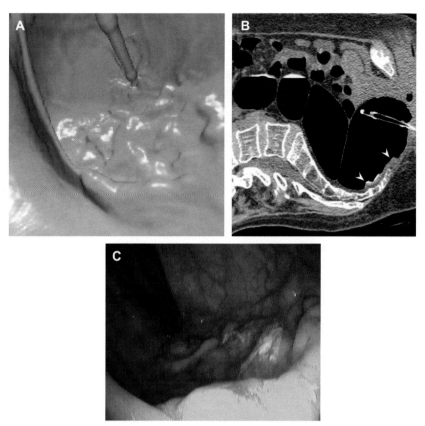

*Fig. 7.* Carpet lesion (villous adenoma) detected at CTC screening. (*A*) 3D endoluminal CTC image shows a large but relatively subtle lobulated mass carpeting a large portion of the distal rectum. (*B*) 2D sagittal CTC image confirms a flat soft tissue mass involving the posterior rectum (*arrowheads*). Optimal distention is critical for detecting such lesions. (*C*) Digital photograph from optical colonoscopy confirms a large, lobulated carpet lesion extending to the anorectal junction. This benign villous adenoma was removed by surgical excision with a transanal approach.

among the MPR views, tends to underestimate polyp size, and the 3D endoluminal view can overestimate polyp size. Therefore, the authors have found it useful to take both measurements into account before deciding on a final value [31]. In the future, polyp volume assessment may play a more prominent role because it is a better indicator of the actual soft tissue mass present and is more sensitive in detecting interval change [32]. In addition to linear size measurement, the segmental location, polyp morphology (pedunculated, sessile, or flat), and diagnostic confidence score for each polyp are recorded. The diagnostic confidence score can provide useful information for the gastroenterologist and for program quality assurance [33]. The authors work closely with their gastroenterology colleagues, particularly with regard to same-day polypectomies. This "one-stop shop" capability assures complete screening with a single bowel preparation, which greatly enhances patient satisfaction and compliance. The authors provide the

colonoscopist with digital images, including the polyp location on the 3D map, a variety of 3D endoluminal projections, and 2D MPR images of the polyp(s) (see Fig. 1). Any polyps located behind a fold are mentioned specifically, because these are more easily missed at colonoscopy [34].

The CTC study is considered negative if no polyps are identified or only potential diminutive lesions ($\leq 5$ mm) are seen. There are a number of reasons why possible diminutive lesions at CTC should not be noted. Most importantly, these findings are not clinically relevant, and their specific mention may raise undue anxiety in patients and referring physicians [1,28,35]. Furthermore, most such "lesions" detected at CTC cannot be found at subsequent colonoscopy, representing either CTC false positives or colonoscopic false negatives. To avoid any confusion or false pretenses, the authors include the following statement in all of their CTC reports: "Note: CT colonography is not intended for the detection of diminutives polyps ($\leq 5$ mm), the presence or

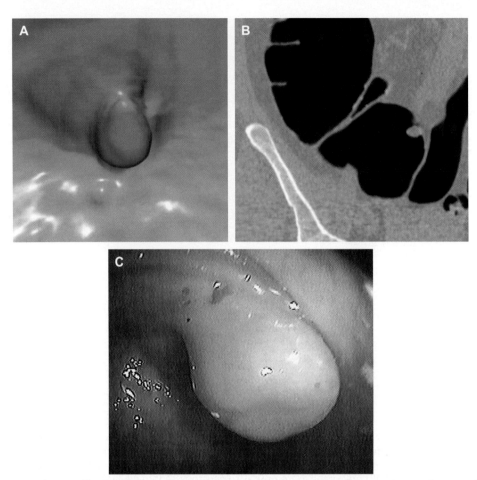

*Fig. 8.* Inverted appendiceal stump simulating a polyp. (*A*) 3D endoluminal CTC image shows a large sessile polypoid lesion in the cecum. (*B*) 2D coronal CTC image shows that the lesion is composed of soft tissue but is located in the expected region of prior appendectomy. Although an inverted appendiceal stump was questioned, the patient was sent for same-day optical colonoscopy because a neoplastic polyp could not be excluded confidently. (*C*) Digital photograph from optical colonoscopy confirms an inverted appendiceal stump. Biopsies showed only normal colonic mucosa. Lesion location and surgical history can avoid the need for colonoscopy referral in most but not all cases.

absence of which will not change the clinical management of the patient." For negative CTC studies, the authors currently recommend repeat colorectal screening in approximately 5 years.

After screening more than 4,000 asymptomatic adults at UWHC, the authors' CTC test-positive rate at the 6-mm threshold has remained steady at about 12% [29]. Because of a significant decrease in false positives, this positivity rate is much lower than the 30% rate predicted from the screening trial [1]. Importantly, however, this increase in specificity does not seem to come at the cost of decreased sensitivity. In fact, a direct comparison of CTC and optical colonoscopy programs at UWHC shows that the detection rates for advanced adenomas are similar [30], even though fewer than 10% of patients screened by CTC undergo subsequent

invasive colonoscopy. In addition, the number of polypectomies performed to yield the same number of advanced adenomas is almost an order of magnitude less than with primary CTC than with primary optical colonoscopy. This comparison is strong evidence that CTC is almost an effective and efficient minimally invasive filter for finding the true target lesion of colorectal cancer screening.

### Diagnostic pitfalls

A number of potential diagnostic pitfalls in CTC interpretation must be recognized [3]. Some pitfalls present more of a problem on 2D evaluation, such as prominent or complex folds (Fig. 5), diverticular fold thickening, and shifting of pedunculated polyps. Others are more of an issue on 3D, such as annular masses, submucosal or extrinsic lesions, and impacted diverticula. With a biphasic interpretive approach, most of these pitfalls are avoided easily because of the complementary nature of the 2D and 3D displays.

With the use of oral contrast tagging, residual stool is now a rare cause of a false-positive examination, in the authors' experience. One additional potential pitfall related to tagging is the tendency for soft tissue polyps to retain a thin surface coating of adherent contrast [36]. This contrast etching actually serves as a beacon for detection. Focal luminal collapse remains the leading cause of nondiagnostic segmental evaluation, because neither 2D nor 3D can properly exclude significant lesions in such areas. Fortunately, this situation has also become quite rare with the authors' current distention protocol. Advanced diverticular disease is responsible for a number of potential pitfalls, including luminal collapse, fold thickening, and impacted diverticula (Fig. 6). With the authors' biphasic 3D/2D interpretive approach, the overall accuracy for polyp detection in these segments does not seem to be adversely affected, however [37].

Flat lesions are less conspicuous and therefore are more challenging to detect at CTC. Important flat lesions are rarely missed with the authors' approach, however, and they generally do not seem to represent a significant drawback to CTC screening in the United States [38,39]. Carpet lesions, despite their large linear dimensions, can be relatively subtle on CTC but also are generally detectable with the authors' biphasic interpretive approach and optimal technique (Fig. 7). In the author's experience, true carpet lesions are rare but typically are large and often prove to be villous adenomas, whereas smaller flat lesions under 3 cm tend to be non-neoplastic hyperplastic lesions. Most polyps of significant size missed by the authors' CTC approach turn out to be nonadenomatous in nature (predominately hyperplastic), even though they are significantly outnumbered by adenomas at this size [40]. This unintended decrease in CTC sensitivity for nonadenomatous lesions is fortuitous, because they probably lack malignant potential. An isolated thickened fold can present a diagnostic challenge at CTC but, in the authors' experience, these rarely if ever represent significant pathology if they are smooth and uniform appearing on the 3D endoluminal view. Other pitfalls that the authors have encountered on a number of occasions relate to inverted appendiceal stumps (Fig. 8), submucosal vascular blebs, the ileocecal valve (Fig. 9), and the rectal catheter [23,25,41–43].

## Summary

Many disparate facets of a CTC screening program must be addressed properly to achieve patient satisfaction, support from referring clinicians, and overall clinical success. With continued improvements in bowel preparation, colonic distention, and CTC interpretation, the initial results of CTC screening at UWHC have greatly exceeded the authors' original expectations based on the data from the earlier screening trial. Some of the lessons the authors learned during the initial phase of program set-up need not be repeated by other groups instituting similar programs. When widespread third-party reimbursement for CTC screening arrives, this examination could become a major component of

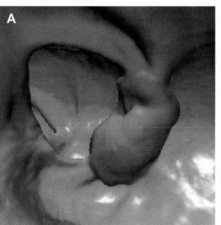 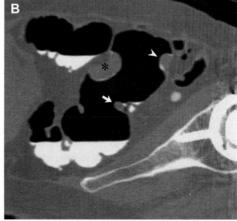

*Fig. 9.* Adenocarcinoma simulating the ileocecal valve on 3D. (*A*) 3D endoluminal CTC image shows a cecal mass that mimics the appearance of a prominent ileocecal valve. (*B*) On the 2D sagittal CTC image the lesion (*asterisk*) is located opposite the valve (*arrow*). A second cecal soft tissue lesion is also present (*arrowhead*). Both masses proved to be adenocarcinoma at pathologic evaluation.

many radiology practices. As such, CTC screening ultimately could have a tremendous positive impact on colorectal cancer screening and prevention.

## References

[1] Pickhardt PJ, Choi JR, Hwang I, et al. CT virtual colonoscopy to screen for colorectal neoplasia in asymptomatic adults. N Engl J Med 2003;349: 2191–200.

[2] Pickhardt PJ, Taylor AJ, Kim DH, et al. Screening for colorectal neoplasia with CT colonography: initial experience from the first year of coverage by third-party payers. Radiology 2006;241: 417–25.

[3] Pickhardt PJ. Screening CT colonography (virtual colonoscopy): technique & interpretation. AJR Am J Roentgenol, in press.

[4] Pickhardt PJ, Taylor AJ, Johnson GL, et al. Building a CT colonography program: necessary ingredients for reimbursement and clinical success. Radiology 2005;235:17–20.

[5] Pickhardt PJ. Virtual colonoscopy for primary screening: the future is now. Minerva Chir 2005; 60:139–50.

[6] Markowitz GS, Stokes MB, Radhakrishnan J, et al. Acute phosphate nephropathy following oral sodium phosphate bowel purgative: an underrecognized cause of chronic renal failure. J Am Soc Nephrol 2005;16:3389–96.

[7] Kim DH, Pickhardt PJ, Hinshaw JL, et al. Prospective blinded trial comparing 45-ml and 90-ml doses of oral sodium phosphate for bowel preparation prior to CT colonography. J Comput Assist Tomogr 2007;31:53–8.

[8] Pickhardt PJ, Choi JR. Electronic cleansing and stool tagging in CT colonography: advantages and pitfalls encountered with primary three-dimensional evaluation. AJR Am J Roentgenol 2003;181:799–805.

[9] Miller MT, Pickhardt PJ, Franaszek M, et al. Assessment of bowel opacification on oral contrast-enhanced CT colonography: multi-institutional trial [abstract]. Presented at the 2004 Society of Gastrointestinal Radiologists meeting. Scottsdale (AZ), March 7–12, 2004.

[10] Summers RM, Franaszek M, Miller MT, et al. Computer-aided detection of polyps in oral contrast-enhanced CT colonography. AJR Am J Roentgenol 2005;184:105–8.

[11] Pickhardt PJ. The incidence of colonic perforation at CT colonography: review of the existing data and the implications for screening of asymptomatic adults. Radiology 2006;239:313–6.

[12] Shinners TJ, Pickhardt PJ, Taylor AJ, et al. Patient-controlled room air insufflation versus automated carbon dioxide delivery for CT colonography. AJR Am J Roentgenol 2006;186: 1491–6.

[13] Summers RM, Yao J, Pickhardt PJ, et al. Computed tomographic virtual colonoscopy computer-aided polyp detection in a screening population. Gastroenterology 2005;129:1832–44.

[14] Choi M, Taylor AJ, VonBerge JL, et al. Can the CT scout reliably assess for adequate colonic distention at CT colonography [abstract]? Presented at the 2005 American Roentgen Ray Society meeting. New Orleans (LA), May 15–20, 2005.

[15] Brenner DJ, Georgsson MA. Mass screening with CT colonography: should radiation exposure be of concern? Gastroenterology 2005;129: 328–37.

[16] Pickhardt PJ. Virtual colonoscopy: issues related to primary screening. Eur Radiol 2005;15(Suppl 4):D133–7.

[17] Pickhardt PJ, Taylor AJ. Extracolonic findings identified in asymptomatic adults at screening CT colonography. AJR Am J Roentgenol 2006; 186:718–28.

[18] Johnson CD, Harmsen WS, Wilson LA, et al. Prospective blinded evaluation of computed tomographic colonography for screen detection of colorectal polyps. Gastroenterology 2003;125: 311–9.

[19] Cotton PB, Durkalski VL, Pineau BC, et al. Computed tomographic colonography (virtual colonoscopy): a multicenter comparison with standard colonoscopy for detection of colorectal neoplasia. JAMA 2004;291:1713–9.

[20] Rockey DC, Paulsen EK, Niedzwiecki D, et al. Analysis of air contrast barium enema, computed tomographic colonography, and colonoscopy: prospective comparison. Lancet 2005;365:305–11.

[21] Cash BD, Kim C, Cullen P, et al. Accuracy of computed tomographic colonography for colorectal cancer screening in asymptomatic individuals [abstract]. Presented at the Digestive Disease Week 2006 annual meeting. Los Angeles (CA), May 20–25, 2006. p. 473.

[22] Pickhardt PJ. Three-dimensional endoluminal CT colonography (virtual colonoscopy): comparison of three commercially available systems. AJR Am J Roentgenol 2003;181:1599–606.

[23] Pickhardt PJ. Differential diagnosis of polypoid lesions seen at CT colonography (virtual colonoscopy). Radiographics 2004;24:1535–59.

[24] Pickhardt PJ, Taylor AJ, Gopal DV. Surface visualization at 3D endoluminal CT colonography: degree of coverage and implications for polyp detection. Gastroenterology 2006;130:1582–7.

[25] Pickhardt PJ. Translucency rendering in 3D endoluminal CT colonography: a useful tool for increasing polyp specificity and decreasing interpretation time. AJR Am J Roentgenol 2004; 183:429–36.

[26] Franaszek M, Summers RM, Pickhardt PJ, et al. Assessment of obscured colonic surface in CT colonography [abstract]. Presented at the 2004 Radiological Society of North America scientific assembly. Chicago, November 28–December 3, 2004.

[27] Zalis ME, Barish MA, Choi JR, et al. for the Working Group on Virtual Colonoscopy. CT colonography

reporting and data system: a consensus proposal. Radiology 2005;236:3–9.

[28] Pickhardt PJ. CT colonography (virtual colonoscopy) for primary colorectal screening: challenges facing clinical implementation. Abdom Imaging 2005;30:1–4.

[29] Pickhardt PJ, Kim DH, Taylor AJ, et al. CT colonography reporting and data system (C-RADS): prospective categorization for screening in 2,501 patients [abstract]. Presented at the 2006 Radiological Society of North America scientific assembly. Chicago, November 26–December 1, 2006.

[30] Kim DH, Pickhardt PJ, Taylor AJ, et al. Advanced adenomas identified at colorectal screening: comparison between CT colonography and optical colonoscopy programs [abstract]. Presented at the 2006 Radiological Society of North America scientific assembly. Chicago, November 26–December 1, 2006.

[31] Pickhardt PJ, Lee AD, McFarland EG, et al. Linear polyp measurement at CT colonography: in vitro and in vivo comparison of two-dimensional and three-dimensional displays. Radiology 2005;236:872–8.

[32] Pickhardt PJ, Lehman VT, Winter TC, et al. Comparison of polyp volume versus linear size measurement at CT colonography: implications for noninvasive surveillance of unresected colorectal lesions. AJR Am J Roentgenol 2006;186:1605–10.

[33] Pickhardt PJ, Choi JR, Nugent PA, et al. The effect of diagnostic confidence on the probability of optical colonoscopic confirmation for potential polyps detected at CT colonography: prospective assessment in 1339 asymptomatic adults. AJR Am J Roentgenol 2004;183:1661–5.

[34] Pickhardt PJ, Nugent PA, Mysliwiec PA, et al. Location of adenomas missed at optical colonoscopy. Ann Intern Med 2004;141:352–9.

[35] Bond JH. Clinical relevance of the small colorectal polyp. Endoscopy 2001;33:454–7.

[36] O'Connor SD, Summers RM, Yao J, et al. Oral contrast adherence to polyps on CT colonography. J Comput Assist Tomogr 2006;30:51–7.

[37] Sanford MS, Pickhardt PJ. Diagnostic performance of primary 3-dimensional computed tomography colonography in the setting of colonic diverticular disease. Clin Gastroenterol Hepatol 2006;4:1039–47.

[38] Pickhardt PJ, Nugent PA, Choi JR, et al. Flat colorectal lesions in asymptomatic adults: implications for screening with CT virtual colonoscopy. AJR Am J Roentgenol 2004;183:1343–7.

[39] Pickhardt PJ. High-magnification chromoscopic colonoscopy: caution needs to be exercised before changing screening policy [reply]. AJR Am J Roentgenol 2006;186:577–8.

[40] Pickhardt PJ, Choi JR, Hwang I, et al. Nonadenomatous polyps at CT colonography: prevalence, size distribution, and detection rates. Radiology 2004;232:784–90.

[41] Prout TM, Taylor AJ, Pickhardt PJ. Inverted appendiceal stumps simulating large pedunculated polyps at screening CT colonography. AJR Am J Roentgenol 2006;186:535–8.

[42] Lee AD, Pickhardt PJ, Gopal DV, et al. Venous malformations mimicking multiple mucosal polyps at screening CT colonography. AJR Am J Roentgenol 2006;186:1113–5.

[43] Pickhardt PJ, Choi JR. Adenomatous polyp obscured by small-caliber rectal catheter at CT colonography: a rare diagnostic pitfall. AJR Am J Roentgenol 2005;184:1581–3.

RADIOLOGIC
CLINICS
OF NORTH AMERICA

Radiol Clin N Am 45 (2007) 377–387

# MR Colonography

Sonja Kinner, MD[a], Thomas C. Lauenstein, MD[a,b,*]

- Techniques of MR colonography
- Indications of MR colonoscopy and clinical outcome
  *Detection of colorectal masses*
  *Inflammatory bowel disease*
- *Patients with incomplete optical colonoscopy*
  *Other indications*
- Acceptance of MR colonography
- Virtual colonoscopy: MR imaging or CT?
- References

Optical colonoscopy has been considered the modality of choice for the assessment of colonic pathologies including the detection of colorectal masses and the depiction of bowel wall inflammation [1,2]. It is an accurate tool providing the ability to gather tissue samples simultaneously for further histopathologic characterization. Despite its great diagnostic value, there are several drawbacks to conventional endoscopy. Because of its invasive character and procedural pain coupled with the rigors of preparatory bowel cleansing, patients' acceptance is limited [3,4]. This lack of acceptance is underlined by the fact that only moderate patient participation is observed in screening programs, even if access to colonoscopy is free of charge [5,6]. Furthermore, there is a small but existing risk of bowel wall perforation [7]. Endoscopic procedures can be incomplete because of colonic stenoses or elongated bowel loops, which may be found in up to 26% of all patients [8,9]. Thus, there has been a need to develop alternative diagnostic procedures to visualize the large bowel.

Virtual colonography (VC) was first introduced by Vining and colleagues [10] in 1994 and has evolved during the last decade as a promising alternative to optical endoscopy. The concept of VC is based on the acquisition of cross-sectional images of the abdomen using either CT or MR imaging. Because of the administration of either liquid or gasiform distending media, the colonic wall can be assessed either on the acquired source data or on virtual endoscopic reformations [11,12]. VC overcomes some of the disadvantages of optical colonoscopy. The entire large bowel can be depicted even in the presence of stenotic lesions or elongated bowel segments. The data sets can be assessed in a multiplanar reformation mode on a postprocessing workstation, which enables the display of the colon from any desired angle. This type of multiplanar reformation analysis depicts the colonic wall, the colonic lumen, and all the surrounding abdominal morphology. Hence, analysis is not limited to the bowel itself. All adjacent abdominal structures can be assessed, so colonic lesions can be located more accurately [13]. Finally, most patients prefer VC to conventional endoscopy and would choose VC if both modalities were accessible [14–16]. Because of higher clinical availability of scanners and economic rationales, most VC approaches so far have focused on CT colonoscopy (CTC). MR colonography (MRC) has evolved as an alternative method that has several advantages over CTC,

[a] Department of Radiology and Neuroradiology, University Hospital, Hufelandstrasse 55, 45122 Essen, Germany
[b] Department of Radiology, Emory University Hospital, The Emory Clinic, 1365 Clifton Road, Bldg A, Suite AT-627, Atlanta, GA 30322, USA
* Corresponding author. Department of Radiology, The Emory Clinic, 1365 Clifton Road, Bldg A, Suite AT-627, Atlanta, GA 30322.
*E-mail address:* tlauens@emory.edu (T.C. Lauenstein).

doi:10.1016/j.rcl.2007.03.004

including the lack of ionizing radiation, better soft tissue contrast, and the use of non-nephrotoxic intravenous contrast compounds.

## Techniques of MR colonography

There are several prerequisites for MRC. Bowel purgation must be performed in a way similar to that required for optical colonoscopy. Different substances for bowel purgation are available [17], and the cleansing process should be started the evening before the MR scan. Before the examination patients must be screened for general contraindications to MR imaging including the presence of metallic implants or severe claustrophobia. Hip prostheses, which generally are not considered a contraindication to MR imaging, can result in considerable artifacts in the pelvis, thereby impeding acquisition of an image of the sigmoid colon and rectum that has adequate diagnostic quality. Thus, these patients should be excluded. For adequate visualization of the large bowel, two main issues must be considered.

First, because most colonic loops are collapsed in their physiologic state, the large bowel needs to be distended to allow a reliable assessment of the bowel wall. Otherwise, nondistended colonic segments may mimic bowel wall thickening and lead to a misinterpretation of inflammation or even colorectal malignancy. Furthermore, smaller lesions, such as colorectal polyps, may be missed. To assure sufficient distension, the rectal administration of water, water-based fluids, air, or carbon dioxide has been proposed [18–21]. Furthermore, spasmolytic agents (eg, 20 mg scopolamine or 1 mg glucagon) should be administered intravenously to help obviate bowel spasms, minimize artifacts caused by bowel motion, and provide greater bowel distension [22].

Second, high contrast between the bowel wall and bowel lumen is crucial for reliable visualization of pathology arising from the colonic wall. The contrast mechanisms depend on the MR sequences as well as on the composition of the rectal enema. There are two different types of contrast: a "bright-lumen" MRC with a dark-appearing bowel wall, and a "dark-lumen" MRC with a signal-intense colonic wall. Bright-lumen MRC images can be obtained by acquiring T2-weighted images in conjunction with a rectal enema consisting of water (Fig. 1), or by collecting T1-weighted data after the administration of a gadolinium-based rectal enema. Dark-lumen MRC images can be obtained by the rectal administration of water, air, or carbon dioxide in conjunction with an acquisition of contrast-enhanced T1-weighted data (Fig. 2).

Similar to contrast-enhanced three-dimensional (3D) MR angiography, MRC is based on the principles of ultra-fast imaging. Each sequence must be acquired under breath-hold conditions. Hence, the use of an appropriate hardware system is mandatory. In the past most MRC techniques have been applied using 1.5-Tesla (T) scanners equipped with strong gradient systems. Recent studies have proven feasibility of MRC on 3.0-T systems [23,24]. After the placement of a rectal tube or a Foley catheter, the authors suggest the administration of approximately 2000 to 2500 mL of warm water using hydrostatic pressure. The filling procedure should be stopped if the patient complains about discomfort such as abdominal cramps or pain. Non–slice-select sequences providing an update image every 2 to 3 seconds can be acquired during the filling process to ensure an adequate distension.

The patient can be scanned in either prone or supine position depending on the patient's preference. For signal reception, a combination of two flex surface coils should be used to assure the coverage of the entire abdomen and pelvis. After obtaining

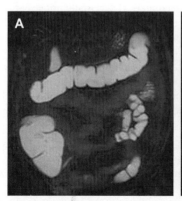 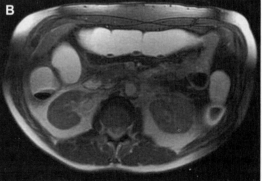

*Fig. 1.* Bright-lumen MRC approach. After a rectal enema consisting of water, the bowel lumen shows high signal intensity on (*A*) single-shot T2-weighted images and (*B*) TrueFISP (Siemens Medical Solutions, Erlangen, Germany) images, whereas the bowel wall appears dark.

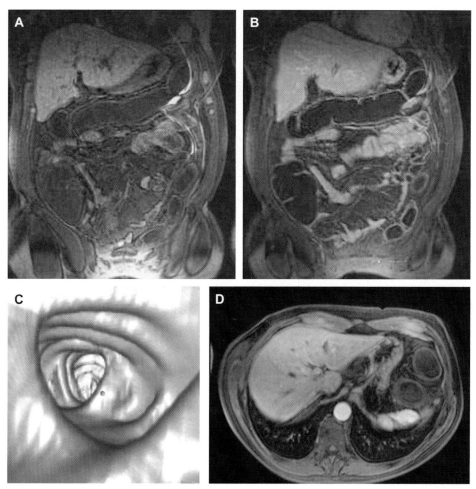

*Fig. 2.* Dark-lumen MRC with T1-weighted images (*A*) before and (*B*) after intravenous gadolinium. (*C*) The 3D data sets can be displayed as a virtual endoscopic view. (*D*) Images also should be collected in an arterial phase of the upper abdomen to allow a detailed assessment of liver and pancreas.

a localizer sequence, the authors propose the acquisition of two-dimensional and/or 3D fast imaging with steady-state precession (FISP) sequences. Different vendor-specific names for these sequences have been introduced: TrueFISP (Siemens Medical Solutions, Erlangen, Germany), Balanced Fast Field Echo (Philips Medical Systems, Best, the Netherlands), and FIESTA (General Electric Medical Systems, Milwaukee, Wisconsin). Image features are characterized by a mixture of both T1 and T2 contrast, creating a homogenous bright signal of the colonic lumen filled with water. One of the main advantages of this type of sequence is its relative insensitivity to motion, which might be especially helpful in patients unable to hold their breath. These data should be collected without fat suppression, because the technique allows good visualization of the colon itself and also of mesenteric structures (eg, mesenteric lymph nodes). In addition, the authors find the acquisition of coronal and axial single-shot T2-weighted sequences with fat saturation helpful. These sequences are essential for the depiction of edema in or adjacent to the bowel wall (Fig. 3) and can be used to distinguish active from chronic inflammatory processes. Finally, T1-weighted MR imaging should be performed in conjunction with the intravenous administration of paramagnetic contrast. After a first precontrast T1-weighted 3D gradient echo data set, paramagnetic contrast should be administered intravenously at a dosage of 0.1 to 0.2 mmol/kg. The 3D acquisition should be repeated in the coronal plane at 70 seconds and 120 seconds following intravenous contrast administration. The authors also recommend taking advantage of the contrast injection and the relatively long delay before the first contrast-enhanced coronal 3D data set to image the liver in an arterial phase (eg, after a contrast delay of

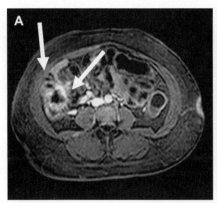 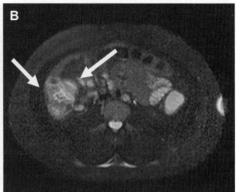

*Fig. 3.* Dark-lumen MRC in a patient who has colitis. (*A*) Contrast-enhanced T1-weighted image shows increased contrast enhancement of the ascending colon (*arrows*). (*B*) On the fat-suppressed T2-weighted image, adjacent edema can be depicted (*arrows*) a sensitive indicator of active inflammatory disease.

20 seconds) using the same sequence in axial plane (see Fig. 2D). This sequence should be collected again in the axial plane at 180 seconds to provide information of an equilibrium contrast phase. All sequence parameters are listed in Table 1. A summary of data acquisition is shown in Table 2.

After the scan, all data sets should be analyzed on a postprocessing workstation. The authors recommend interpreting the contrast-enhanced 3D T1-weighted images in a multiplanar reformation mode. Thus, the radiologist can scroll through the data set in all three orthogonal planes. When a colorectal lesion is seen on the contrast-enhanced sequence, it must be compared with the precontrast T1-weighted image. Hence, a safe differentiation between residual stool particles and real colorectal lesions is possible: colorectal lesions always show a strong contrast enhancement (Fig. 4), whereas residual stool never does (Fig. 5). In a second step, the FISP sequences and T2-weighted single-shot images need to be analyzed. In addition, special software tools can provide virtual endoscopic views of the colonic wall, and virtual a fly-through can be performed. The fly-through should be performed in both an antegrade and retrograde direction [25] so that even small lesions can be detected more accurately. Furthermore, 3D depth perception improves the radiologist's ability to distinguish haustra from colorectal masses.

## Indications of MR colonoscopy and clinical outcome

### *Detection of colorectal masses*

Several trials have assessed the ability of MRC to detect colorectal lesions (Table 3). First approaches were based mainly on bright-lumen techniques using a gadolinium-based rectal enema [26–28]. Pappalardo and colleagues [26] examined 70 consecutive patients initially referred for conventional colonoscopy. The diagnostic ability of MRC for the detection of colonic lesions was determined and compared with optical colonoscopy. MRC achieved a high accuracy, with 93% sensitivity and 97% specificity for the detection of colorectal lesions independent on their size. Furthermore, even a higher total number of polyps were detected by MRC in this trial, because additional lesions were found in regions not accessible by optical colonoscopy. A trial by Luboldt and colleagues [27] demonstrated that diagnostic accuracy of MRC was highly dependant on polyp size: although most polyps smaller than 5 mm were not detected

*Table 1:*   **Sequence parameters for MR colonography**

| | 2D FISP without fat suppression | 2D Single-shot T2-weighted with fat suppression | 3D T1-weighted GRE with fat suppression |
|---|---|---|---|
| TR [ms] | 3.7 | 676 | 1.9 |
| TE [ms] | 1.9 | 100 | 3.9 |
| Flip [°] | 60 | 90 | 10 |
| Slice thickness | 4–5 mm | 6–7 mm | 2 mm |

*Abbreviations:* FISP, fast imaging with steady-state precession; GRE, gradient recalled echo; TE, echo time; TR, repitition time; 2D, two-dimensional.

**Table 2:** Features of MR sequences and their information content

| Sequence | Orientation | Contrast delay | Features |
|---|---|---|---|
| 2D FISP without fat suppression | axial/coronal | – | Depiction of anatomy Assessment of mesenteries Relatively insensitive to motion |
| 2D single-shot T2-weighted with fat suppression | axial/coronal | – | Assessment of bowel wall edema |
| 3D T1-weighted GRE with fat suppression | coronal | 0 s, 70 s, 120 s | Assessment of colonic masses and inflammation Perfusion information |
| 3D T1-weighted GRE with fat suppression | axial | 20 s, 180 s | Display of liver of other parenchymal organs in abdomen and pelvis |

*Abbreviations:* FISP, fast imaging with steady-state precession; GRE, gradient recalled echo; 2D, two-dimensional.

by MRC, the sensitivity for the detection of polyps larger than 10 mm was greater than 90%.

A further improvement was the introduction of dark-lumen MRC concepts. The diagnostic accuracy of bright- and dark-lumen MRC was compared in a study performed in 37 patients suspected of having colorectal lesions [29]. Warm tap water was used to distend the large bowel. The detection rate of

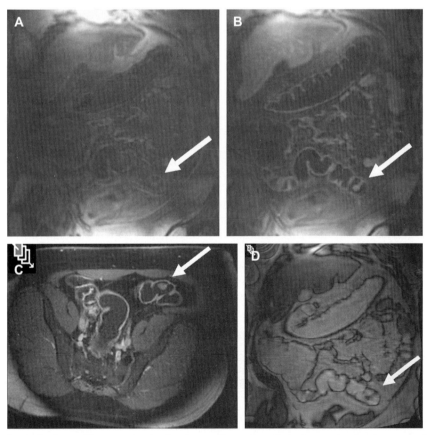

*Fig. 4.* A patient who has a 10-mm polyp in the descending colon. Note the contrast enhancement comparing the pre- (*A*) and post-gadolinium enhanced (*B*) T1-weighted coronal images (*arrows*). The lesion can also be depicted on T1-weighted axial post contrast (*C, arrow*), and TrueFISP (Siemens Medical Solutions, Erlangen, Germany) bright-lumen (*D, arrow*).

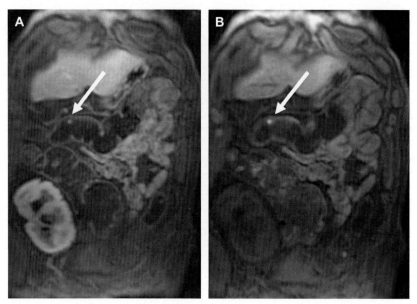

*Fig. 5.* Residual stool may mimic colonic lesions on T1-weighted post-contrast scans (*A, arrow*). However, due to lack of enhancement in comparison to pre-contrast scans (*B, arrow*), fecal material can be accurately differentiated from polyps.

colorectal masses and inflammatory lesions was assessed separately for T1-weighted data with and without intravenous contrast (dark-lumen MRC) and FISP sequences (bright-lumen MRC). Furthermore, the image quality of both sequence types was analyzed. Subsequent conventional colonoscopy served as a standard of reference. The overall sensitivity of dark-lumen MRC for the depiction of polyps was 79%. Only four polyps smaller than 5 mm were missed. Specificity, however, was as high as 100%, because residual stool could be differentiated from colorectal masses reliably. The sensitivity for bright-lumen MRC, however, was only 68.4% because two additional polyps (7 and 8 mm) could not be detected. Because of the inability to distinguish residual stool particles from real colorectal masses, there were false-positive results in five patients. The image quality of the FISP sequences was superior to that of T1-weighted imaging, however, because there were fewer motion artifacts.

Thus, both T1-weighted and FISP imaging should be included in a comprehensive MRC protocol.

In a recent trial, dark-lumen MRC was compared prospectively with optical endoscopy in a larger cohort of 100 patients [30]. All subjects underwent bowel purgation for MR imaging and colonoscopy. MR data collection and evaluation were based mainly on pre- and postgadolinium T1-weighted data. With optical colonoscopy 107 colorectal masses were detected in 49 patients. The sensitivity of MRC for adenomas on a per-lesion basis was 84% for polyps between 6 and 9 mm in diameter and 100% for lesions larger than 10 mm. On a per-patient analysis, the overall sensitivity for the detection of colorectal masses was 90% with 96% specificity. Similar results were published by Ajaj and colleagues [31]. One hundred twenty-two subjects suspected of having colorectal disease underwent MR imaging and subsequent conventional endoscopy. Although none of the polyps smaller than

*Table 3:* **Diagnostic accuracy of MRC for the detection of colorectal masses in comparison to optical colonoscopy**

| Author | Year | Patients (n) | Polyps 5–10 mm (% detected) | Polyps > 10 mm (% detected) |
|---|---|---|---|---|
| Pappalardo [26] | 2000 | 70 | 97 | 100 |
| Luboldt [27] | 2000 | 132 | 61 | 94 |
| Hartmann [30] | 2006 | 100 | 84 | 100 |
| Ajaj [31] | 2003 | 120 | 89 | 100 |

5 mm could be visualized by MRC, 16 of 18 lesions between 5 and 10 mm were detected correctly. Furthermore, all polyps larger than 10 mm and nine carcinomas were depicted correctly. Thus, one major drawback of MRC is its inability to detect accurately colorectal lesions smaller than 5 mm. The importance of this limitation is controversial, because small polyps are not prone to malignant degeneration but remain stable over a time range of 3 to 5 years [32]. Most studies evaluating MRC were performed in high-risk cohorts. Few data are available on MRC as a screening tool. In a recent trial, Kuehle and colleagues [33] investigated more than 300 screening patients older than 50 years who did not have an increased risk profile for colorectal cancer. MRC data were analyzed for the presence of colorectal masses and compared with optical colonoscopy findings. Adenomatous polyps larger than 5 mm were detected with a sensitivity of 74%, which increased to 93% for lesions larger than 10 mm. The specificity of MRC for the detection of colorectal lesions was 93%.

### Inflammatory bowel disease

MRC has been used successfully for the diagnosis and characterization of inflammatory bowel disease (IBD) including ulcerative colitis and Crohn's disease. Although endoscopy in conjunction with biopsy is still considered the standard procedure for the evaluation of IBD [34,35], several studies have investigated the use of MR imaging for detecting and quantifying IBD [36–39]. Schreyer and colleagues [40] assessed the use of MRC for the depiction of IBD. Although MRC failed to depict the most subtle inflammatory changes, it revealed severe inflammation with high accuracy. It often has been discussed whether MRC can assess the grade of inflammation activity. Ajaj and colleagues [38] focused on this issue, using MR imaging to examine 23 patients suspected of having IBD of the large bowel. Inflammatory changes of the colonic wall were documented and quantified according to four criteria: bowel wall thickness, bowel wall contrast enhancement, loss of haustral folds, and presence of perifocal lymph nodes. A MRC-based inflammation score was determined and correlated with histopathologic findings. In this study, more than 90% of the colonic segments with IBD changes were diagnosed correctly and categorized as mildly, moderately, or severely inflamed. The evaluation of contrast enhancement patterns to determine the grade of inflammation has been controversial. Florie and colleagues [41] examined 48 patients who had Crohn's disease. They found that the enhancement ratio of bowel wall after intravenous administration of gadodiamide and bowel wall thickness are only weak-to-moderate indicators of the severity of Crohn's disease. Maccioni and colleagues [42] described the combined analysis of T2-weighted imaging and analysis of contrast enhancement after the intravenous administration of gadolinium. The authors found T2-weighted imaging with fat saturation particularly helpful in providing information about inflammatory activity, because the presence of intra- and perimural edema can be assessed easily (see Fig. 3). Chronic inflammation with fibrotic changes also shows increased contrast enhancement and therefore enhancement patterns should not be used as a single parameter to distinguish active from chronic inflammation.

Another technical consideration is related to the fact that IBD often may affect both the small and large bowel simultaneously. The terminal ileum is the part of the gastrointestinal tract that is affected most often in patients who have Crohn's disease. Furthermore, patients who have ulcerative colitis may show backwash ileitis [43]. Thus, it seems advantageous to visualize the small bowel as well. The small bowel can be visualized by administering oral contrast agents before the MR examination, leading to distension and visualization of small bowel loops (Fig. 6). Narin and colleagues [44] examined 18 patients who had IBD by applying both oral and rectal contrast. T1-weighted data sets were collected before and after intravenous gadolinium administration. The oral ingestion and the rectal application of water allowed assessment of the small bowel and colon in all patients. More inflamed

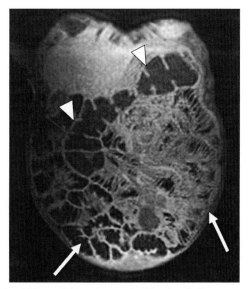

*Fig. 6.* In patients suspected of having inflammatory bowel disease, the authors recommend the administration of oral contrast before MRC. Thus, a simultaneous evaluation of small bowel (*arrows*) and colon (*arrowhead*) is possible.

bowel segments in the colon and terminal ileum were detected by MR imaging than by colonoscopy. Furthermore, eight inflammatory lesions in the jejunum and proximal ileum that had not been endoscopically accessible were found by MR imaging. The depiction of inflammatory processes is not limited to the bowel wall; fistulae and abscesses, which often are not even suspected by endoscopy, can be depicted with MR imaging.

### Patients with incomplete optical colonoscopy

MRC has been shown to provide additional information in patients after incomplete endoscopy [45,46]. There are several reasons why proximal colonic segments might not be accessible by optical endoscopy (eg, presence of stenoses or elongated bowel segments). Water or gasiform distending media, however, can retrogradely pass even high-grade stenoses enabling distension and visualization of prestenotic segments. Hence, MRC has a significantly higher completion rate than optical colonoscopy. Hartmann and colleagues [45] evaluated the impact of MRC in 32 patients who had undergone incomplete optical colonoscopy because of high-grade stenoses, bowel elongation, and patient intolerance. In that trial, all stenoses were identified correctly on the MR data sets. Several polyps detected in the prestenotic bowel segments by MR imaging were proven by subsequent surgery and/or postoperative endoscopy. The impact of MRC in this patient cohort was confirmed by Ajaj and colleagues [46]. In 37 patients who had undergone incomplete endoscopy, the presence of colorectal pathologies was assessed on a segmental basis. Although optical colonoscopy was unable to reach about 50% of all potentially visible segments, 96% of the segments were assessable on MR imaging data sets. Furthermore, all stenotic and poststenotic lesions identified at endoscopy were diagnosed correctly by MRC. Again, MRC provided substantial additional information: five polyps, two colorectal carcinomas, and inflammatory changes in four patients were depicted in prestenotic segments.

### Other indications

Colonic resection is a common procedure for patients who have chronic IBD or colorectal malignancies [47]. Postoperative recurrences at the site of the anastomosis with consecutive stricture are frequent, however. MRC has been assessed as a tool to visualize and characterize anastomoses after colorectal surgery. In a recently published trial 39 patients who had end-to-end-anastomoses after surgical treatment underwent MRC [48]. Contrast-enhanced T1-weighted data were acquired after the rectal administration of water. Criteria for the assessment of the anastomoses included bowel

wall thickening and increased contrast uptake. The site of the anastomosis did not show any suspicious features on MR imaging in 23 patients, and this finding was confirmed by optical colonoscopy in 20 cases. In three patients MR imaging missed mild inflammation. In the remaining 16 patients both MRC and conventional endoscopy detected relevant findings including moderate stenoses of the anastomosis (n = 5), recurrent malignant tumors (n = 2), and inflammation (n = 9). MR imaging data did not show any false-positive findings. Thus, the overall sensitivity and specificity for the assessment of the anastomosis were 84% and 100%, respectively.

Beyond the mere morphologic assessment of the colon, first experimental studies also show a value for functional evaluation of the large bowel. Buhmann and colleagues [49] assessed large bowel motility using functional T2-weighted real-time sequences. Twelve healthy subjects underwent functional MR imaging before and after the administration of motility-modifying substances such as erythromycin. For the motility evaluation, changes in the luminal diameter were assessed at defined locations in the ascending, transverse, and descending colon. It was shown that large bowel motility increased significantly after the administration of erythromycin. Despite these promising initial findings, this technique needs further investigation and refinement to be clinically implemented.

### Acceptance of MR colonography

Beyond diagnostic accuracy, patients' acceptance plays a main role in the impact of a diagnostic tool. Several trials comparing CT VC with optical colonoscopy have shown patients generally prefer the virtual modality [14–16]. Bowel cleansing before virtual or optical colonoscopy has been considered the most inconvenient part of the examination [3,50]. Strategies to obviate bowel cleansing for MRC, such as fecal tagging, might increase acceptance levels of virtual colonoscopy significantly [51,52]. Patients' acceptance of a fecal tagging–based MRC protocol has been compared with optical colonoscopy in a large screening cohort of 284 asymptomatic patients over 50 years of age who underwent both MRC and optical colonoscopy within 4 weeks [53]. MRC was based on a fecal-tagging technique. Patients ingested a solution containing 250 mL diatrizoate meglumine and diatrizoate sodium, barium, and locust bean gum with each main meal starting 2 days before the MR examination. Subsequent optical colonoscopy, however, was performed after bowel cleansing. Patients were asked to evaluate both modalities and different aspects of the examinations. In this trial, no significant difference was noted for the overall acceptance of MRC and optical colonoscopy. This result may be related to the administration of sedatives and analgesics during optical colonoscopy so that perception of discomfort was reduced and the entire procedure was considered less painful. The placement of the rectal tube was rated as the most inconvenient part of the MRC procedure, whereas bowel cleansing was regarded most unpleasant for optical colonoscopy. Beyond the implementation of tagging approaches, investigators should be encouraged to use small tubes or flexible catheters, which distend the bowel adequately [54].

## Virtual colonoscopy: MR imaging or CT?

Only a few trials have focused on the comparative analysis between MRC and CTC. Wesseling and colleagues [23] used a colon phantom with simulated haustrae and polyps between 2 and 8 mm in size. The phantom was scanned using multislice CT and 1.5-T and 3.0-T MR imaging. Although detection rate of polyps smaller than 4 mm was significantly higher for CT colonoscopy, there was no relevant difference for the depiction of larger lesions. In another study 42 patients were examined by both MRC and CTC [55]. MRC was found to be even more sensitive for the depiction of colorectal lesions than CT. The protocol of the underlying trial, however, was tailored in favor of MRC using a fluid enema. Furthermore, data acquisition was performed only by spiral CT. It can be concluded that CT and MR imaging have similar accuracy for the visualization of relevant lesions larger than 6 mm.

Although the use of CTC in the depiction of colorectal lesions seems promising, the future of CT-based VC as a screening method remains uncertain. The associated ionizing radiation raises the possibility of a public health concern [56–59]. The lifetime risk for developing a radiation-induced malignant cancer in a screening population using CT has been estimated to be as high as 1 in 50 patients [59]. Thus, a major advantage of MRC is the lack of exposure to ionizing radiation. Although low-dose protocols for CTC have been applied [60,61], a modality without radiation exposure should be preferred if it provides similar diagnostic accuracy. This issue might be less important in an older population but should be considered particularly when young patients who have IBD are involved. A further argument in favor of MRC is that MR intravenous contrast agents have a more favorable safety profile than CT contrast compounds because they are associated with far fewer anaphylactoid reactions and lack nephrotoxicity [62,63].

## References

[1] Kahi CJ, Rex DK. Screening and surveillance of colorectal cancer. Gastrointest Endosc Clin N Am 2005;15:533–47.

[2] Scholmerich J. Inflammatory bowel disease. Endoscopy 2003;35:164–70.

[3] Akerkar GA, Yer J, Hung, et al. Patient experience and preferences toward colon cancer screening: a comparison of virtual colonoscopy and conventional colonoscopy. Gastrointest Endosc 2001; 54:310–5.

[4] Centers for Disease Control and Prevention (CDC). Trends in screening for colorectal cancer–United States, 1997 and 1999. MMWR Morb Mortal Wkly Rep 2001;50(9):162–6.

[5] Mant D, Fuller A, Northover J, et al. Patient compliance with colorectal cancer screening in general practice. Br J Gen Pract 1992;42:18–20.

[6] Frommer DJ. What's new in colorectal cancer screening? J Gastroenterol Hepatol 1998;13: 528–33.

[7] Dominitz JA, Eisen GM, Baron TH, et al. Complications of colonoscopy. Gastrointest Endosc 2003;57:441–5.

[8] Dafnis G, Granath F, Pahlman L, et al. Patient factors influencing the completion rate in colonoscopy. Dig Liver Dis 2005;37:113–8.

[9] Cirocco WC, Rusin LC. Factors that predict incomplete colonoscopy. Dis Colon Rectum 1995; 389:964–8.

[10] Vining DJ, Gelfand DW, Bechtold RE, et al. Technical feasibility of colon imaging with helical CT and virtual reality. AJR Am J Roentgenol 1994; 162:104.

[11] Geenen RW, Hussain SM, Cademartiri F, et al. CT and MR colonography: scanning techniques, postprocessing, and emphasis on polyp detection. Radiographics 2004;24:e18.

[12] Royster AP, Fenlon HM, Clarke PD, et al. CT colonoscopy of colorectal neoplasms: two-dimensional and three-dimensional virtual-reality techniques with colonoscopic correlation. AJR Am J Roentgenol 1997;169:1237–42.

[13] McFarland EG, Brink JA, Pilgram TK, et al. Spiral CT colonography: reader agreement and diagnostic performance with two- and three-dimensional image-display techniques. Radiology 2001;218: 375–83.

[14] Thomeer M, Bielen D, Vanbeckevoort D, et al. Patient acceptance for CT colonography: what is the real issue? Eur Radiol 2002;12:1410–5.

[15] Svensson MH, Svensson E, Lasson A, et al. Patient acceptance of CT colonography and conventional colonoscopy: prospective comparative study in patients with or suspected of having colorectal disease. Radiology 2002;222:337–45.

[16] Van Gelder RE, Birnie E, Florie J, et al. CT colonography and colonoscopy: assessment of

patient preference in a 5-week follow-up study. Radiology 2004;233:328–37.

[17] Tan JJ, Tjandra JJ. Which is the optimal bowel preparation for colonoscopy—a meta-analysis. Colorectal Dis 2006;8:247–58.

[18] Ajaj W, Lauenstein TC, Pelster G, et al. MR colonography: how does air compare to water for colonic distention? J Magn Reson Imaging 2004; 19:216–21.

[19] Bielen DJ, Bosmans HT, De Wever LL, et al. Clinical validation of high-resolution fast spin-echo MR colonography after colon distention with air. J Magn Reson Imaging 2005;22:400–5.

[20] Lomas DJ, Sood RR, Graves MJ, et al. Colon carcinoma: MR imaging with CO2 enema–pilot study. Radiology 2001;219:558–62.

[21] Luboldt W, Frohlich JM, Schneider N, et al. MR colonography: optimized enema composition. Radiology 1999;212:265–9.

[22] Rogalla P, Lembcke A, Ruckert JC, et al. Spasmolysis at CT colonography: butyl scopolamine versus glucagon. Radiology 2005;236:184–8.

[23] Wessling J, Fischbach R, Borchert A, et al. Detection of colorectal polyps: comparison of multidetector row CT and MR colonography in a colon phantom. Radiology 2006;241:125–31.

[24] Rottgen R, Herzog H, Bogen P, et al. MR colonoscopy at 3.0 T: comparison with 1.5 T in vivo and a colon model. Clin Imaging 2006;30:248–53.

[25] Pickhardt PJ, Taylor AJ, Gopal DV. Surface visualization at 3D endoluminal CT colonography: degree of coverage and implications for polyp detection. Gastroenterology 2006;130:1582–7.

[26] Pappalardo G, Polettini E, Frattaroli FM, et al. Magnetic resonance colonography versus conventional colonoscopy for the detection of colonic endoluminal lesions. Gastroenterology 2000; 119:300–4.

[27] Luboldt W, Bauerfeind P, Wildermuth S, et al. Colonic masses: detection with MR colonography. Radiology 2000;216:383–8.

[28] Saar B, Heverhagen JT, Obst T, et al. Magnetic resonance colonography and virtual magnetic resonance colonoscopy with the 1.0-T system: a feasibility study. Invest Radiol 2000;35:521–6.

[29] Lauenstein TC, Ajaj W, Kuehle CA, et al. Magnetic resonance colonography: comparison of contrast-enhanced three-dimensional vibe with two-dimensional FISP sequences: preliminary experience. Invest Radiol 2005;40:89–96.

[30] Hartmann D, Bassler B, Schilling D, et al. Colorectal polyps: detection with dark-lumen MR colonography versus conventional colonoscopy. Radiology 2006;238:143–9.

[31] Ajaj W, Pelster G, Treichel U, et al. Dark lumen magnetic resonance colonography: comparison with conventional colonoscopy for the detection of colorectal pathology. Gut 2003;52:1738–43.

[32] Villavicencio RT, Rex DK. Colonic adenomas: prevalence and incidence rates, growth rates, and miss rates at colonoscopy. Semin Gastrointest Dis 2000;11:185–93.

[33] Kuehle CA, Langhorst J, Ladd SC, et al. MR colonography without bowel cleansing—a prospective cross-sectional study in a screening population. Gut 2007;[Epub ahead of print].

[34] Fiocca R, Ceppa P. The diagnostic reliability of endoscopic biopsies in diagnosis colitis. J Clin Pathol 2003;56:321–2.

[35] Nahon S, Bouhnik Y, Lavergne-Slove A, et al. Colonoscopy accurately predicts the anatomical severity of colonic Crohn's disease attacks: correlation with findings from colectomy specimens. Am J Gastroenterol 2002;12:3102–7.

[36] Kettritz U, Isaacs K, Warshauer DM, et al. Crohn's disease. Pilot study comparing MRI of the abdomen with clinical evaluation. J Clin Gastroenterol 1995;3:249–53.

[37] Koh DM, Miao Y, Chinn RJ, et al. MR imaging evaluation of the activity of Crohn's disease. AJR Am J Roentgenol 2001;6:1325–32.

[38] Ajaj W, Lauenstein TC, Pelster G, et al. MR colonography for the detection of inflammatory diseases of the large bowel: quantifying the inflammatory activity. Gut 2005;54:257–63.

[39] Schreyer AG, Golder S, Scheibl K, et al. Dark lumen magnetic resonance enteroclysis in combination with MRI colonography for whole bowel assessment in patients with Crohn's disease: first clinical experience. Inflamm Bowel Dis 2005;11:388–94.

[40] Schreyer AG, Rath HC, Kikinis R, et al. Comparison of magnetic resonance imaging colonography with conventional colonoscopy for the assessment of intestinal inflammation in patients with inflammatory bowel disease: a feasibility study. Gut 2005;54:250–6.

[41] Florie J, Wasser MN, Arts-Cieslik K, et al. Dynamic contrast-enhanced MRI of the bowel wall for assessment of disease activity in Crohn's disease. AJR Am J Roentgenol 2006;186:1384–92.

[42] Maccioni F, Bruni A, Viscido A, et al. MR imaging in patients with Crohn disease: value of T2-versus T1-weighted gadolinium-enhanced MR sequences with use of an oral superparamagnetic contrast agent. Radiology 2006;238:517–30.

[43] Gore RM, Balthazar EJ, Ghahremani GG, et al. CT features of ulcerative colitis and Crohn's disease. AJR 1996;167:3–15.

[44] Narin B, Ajaj W, Gohde S, et al. Combined small and large bowel MR imaging in patients with Crohn's disease: a feasibility study. Eur Radiol 2004;14:1535–42.

[45] Hartmann D, Bassler B, Schilling D, et al. Incomplete conventional colonoscopy: magnetic resonance colonography in the evaluation of the proximal colon. Endoscopy 2005;37:816–20.

[46] Ajaj W, Lauenstein TC, Pelster G, et al. MR colonography in patients with incomplete conventional colonoscopy. Radiology 2005;234: 452–9.

[47] Eu KW, Seow-Choen F, Ho JM, et al. Local recurrence following rectal resection for cancer. J R Coll Surg Edinb 1998;43:393–6.

[48] Ajaj W, Goyen M, Langhorst J, et al. MR colonography for the assessment of colonic anastomoses. J Magn Reson Imaging 2006;24:101–7.

[49] Buhmann S, Kirchhoff C, Wielage C, et al. Assessment of large bowel motility by cine magnetic resonance imaging using two different prokinetic agents: a feasibility study. Invest Radiol 2005;40:689–94.

[50] Ristvedt SL, McFarland EG, Weinstock LB, et al. Patient preferences for CT colonography, conventional colonography, and bowel preparation. Am J Gastroenterol 2003;98:578–85.

[51] Lauenstein TC, Goehde SC, Ruehm SG, et al. MR colonography with barium-based fecal tagging: initial clinical experience. Radiology 2002;223: 248–54.

[52] Ajaj W, Lauenstein TC, Schneemann H, et al. Magnetic resonance colonography without bowel cleansing using oral and rectal stool softeners (fecal cracking)–a feasibility study. Eur Radiol 2005;15:2079–87.

[53] Kinner S, Kuehle CA, Langhorst J, et al. MR colonography vs. optical colonoscopy: comparison of patient acceptance in a screening population. European Radiology, accepted for publication.

[54] Taylor SA, Halligan S, Goh V, et al. Optimizing colonic distention for multi-detector row CT colonography: effect of hyoscine butylbromide and rectal balloon catheter. Radiology 2003;229: 99–108.

[55] Haykir R, Karakose S, Karabacakoglu A, et al. Three-dimensional MR and axial CT colonography versus conventional colonoscopy for detection of colon pathologies. World J Gastroenterol 2006;12:2345–50.

[56] Debatin JF, Luboldt W, Bauerfeind P. Virtual colonoscopy in 1999: computed tomography or magnetic resonance imaging? Endoscopy 1999; 31:174–9.

[57] Martin DR, Semelka RC. Health effects of ionising radiation from diagnostic CT. Lancet 2006; 367:1712–4.

[58] National Research Council Committee to Assess Healt Risks from Exposure to Low Levels of Ionizing Radiation. Health risks from exposure to low levels of ionizing radiation: BEIR VII Phase 2. Washington, DC: The National Academies Press; 2006. Available at: http://www.nap.edu/books/030909156X/html.

[59] Brenner DJ, Elliston CD. Estimated radiation risks potentially associated with full-body CT screening. Radiology 2004;232:735–8.

[60] Cohnen M, Vogt C, Beck A, et al. Feasibility of MDCT colonography in ultra-low-dose technique in the detection of colorectal lesions: comparison with high-resolution video colonoscopy. AJR Am J Roentgenol 2004;183:1355–9.

[61] van Gelder RE, Venema HW, Florie J, et al. CT colonography: feasibility of substantial dose reduction—comparison of medium to very low doses in identical patients. Radiology 2004;232: 611–20.

[62] Murphy KJ, Brunberg JA, Cohan RH. Adverse reactions to gadolinium contrast media: a review of 36 cases. AJR Am J Roentgenol 1996;167: 847–9.

[63] Prince MR, Arnoldus C, Frisoli JK. Nephrotoxicity of high-dose gadolinium compared with iodinated contrast. J Magn Reson Imaging 1996;6: 162–6.

RADIOLOGIC
CLINICS
OF NORTH AMERICA

Radiol Clin N Am 45 (2007) 389–394

# Index

*Note:* Page numbers of article titles are in **boldface** type.

doi:10.1016/S0033-8389(07)00038-3

# *Moving?*

## Make sure your subscription moves with you!

To notify us of your new address, find your **Clinics Account Number** (located on your mailing label above your name), and contact customer service at:

E-mail: elspcs@elsevier.com

**800-654-2452** (subscribers in the U.S. & Canada)
**407-345-4000** (subscribers outside of the U.S. & Canada)

Fax number: 407-363-9661

**Elsevier Periodicals Customer Service**
6277 Sea Harbor Drive
Orlando, FL 32887-4800

*To ensure uninterrupted delivery of your subscription, please notify us at least 4 weeks in advance of move.